THE BEHAVIORAL
MANAGEMENT OF THE
CARDIAC PATIENT

Developments in Clinical Psychology

Glenn R. Caddy, series editor
Nova University

THE BEHAVIORAL MANAGEMENT OF THE CARDIAC PATIENT

By
D. G. BYRNE
Department of Psychology
Australian National University
Canberra

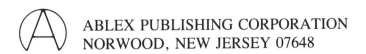
ABLEX PUBLISHING CORPORATION
NORWOOD, NEW JERSEY 07648

Library of Congress Cataloging-in-Publication Data

Byrne, D. G. (Donald Glenn)
  The behavioral management of the cardiac patient.

  (Developments in clinical psychology)
  Includes bibliographies and index.
    1. Heart—Infarction—Psychosomatic aspects.
  2. Coronary heart disease—Psychosomatic aspects.
  3. Behavior therapy. 4. Type A behavior. 5. Heart—
  Diseases—Patients—Rehabilitation. I. Title.
  II. Series. [DNLM: 1. Behavior Therapy. 2. Coronary
  Disease—therapy.   WG 300 B995b]
  RC685.I6B97   1987   616.1'23   87-1324
  ISBN 0-89391-386-3

Ablex Publishing Corporation
355 Chestnut Street
Norwood, New Jersey 07648

Contents

v

CHAPTER 3

PSYCHOLOGICAL RESPONSES TO MYOCARDIAL INFARCTION   36

CHAPTER 4

DETERMINANTS OF OUTCOME FOLLOWING CORONARY HEART DISEASE   58

CHAPTER 5

PSYCHOLOGICAL INTERVENTION FOLLOWING MYOCARDIAL INFARCTION   75

Preface

Heart attack, whether it be given the label coronary heart disease, coronary occlusion, or myocardial infarction, remains a major cause of death and disability in Western, urbanized societies. In many, mortality from heart attack is apparently decreasing, due in part to the early recognition of symptoms and the widespread availability of intensive coronary-care units where constant monitoring of patients in the early stages of their illness can frequently circumvent the effects of the potentially fatal arrhythmias to which such patients are vulnerable. There are less persuasive indications that coronary morbidity is following this trend. It is the survivors of heart attack, the cardiac patients, to whom the substance of this book is directed.

Survivors of heart attack have two broad challenges to overcome. In the short term, while the myocardium remains physiologically sensitive to further damage, they must face the simple challenge of survival. In the longer term, when physiological stability has been restored, they must add to this the challenge of re-establishing participation in their interpersonal, social, and occupational environments, while carrying with them the real or imagined burden of an irreversibly damaged myocardium. In both cases, the process of recovery and rehabilitation is facilitated by the provision of appropriate care. Aside from cardiology, there are few areas in medicine where the conjoined skills of the physician and the clinical psychologist can contribute with such great potential to the care of the patient with life-threatening illness.

The past two decades have seen an enormous output of evidence documenting correlations between psychological and behavioral factors and cardiovascular disease. Emphasis has turned from traditional psychoanalytic views toward a concern with empirical data drawing together concepts as broad as the social environment and as specific as patterns of individual behavior in the search for the mix of factors, both psychological and biological, that must accurately reflect risk of cardiovascular disease. The sheer weight and the emerging consistency of this evidence leave no room for serious doubt that psychological and behavioral factors play causal roles in the several stages leading to heart attack, from the exacerbation of more traditionally accepted risk factors (cigarette smoking, hypertension, and diet), through the deposition of atherosclerotic damage to the coronary arteries to the precipitation of myocardial infarction.

More recently, attention has also turned to the roles that psychological and behavioral factors play in the process of recovery and rehabilitation after heart attack. In this respect, two conclusions are clear. Firstly, significant numbers of patients surviving heart attack respond to that event with emotional distress of sufficient severity to pose, in the short term, a physiological threat to a vulnerable myocardium and, in the long term, a psychological threat to the successful re-establishment of interpersonal and social ties and occupational activities. Secondly, survivors of heart attack may, over a period of time, develop behaviors in response to illness that are at odds with a wholly successful recovery, rehabilitation, or control of further coronary risk.

With this evidence in mind, the potential contribution of psychological and behavioral treatments to the overall management of the cardiac patient is not difficult to see. Indeed, evaluative research assessing the effectiveness of these treatments is increasingly persuasive in suggesting that due attention to the psychological and behavioral needs of the cardiac patient bring about outcome benefits significantly in excess of those to be gained from medical care alone. These studies and their application in clinical practice form the primary substance of the present book.

The book was written to fill the particular needs of the clinical psychologist in a general hospital or community practice for whom the care of the medically ill patient is becoming an increasing responsibility. Its content is obviously of equal importance to physicians, nurses, occupational therapists, and others involved with the day-to-day care of the cardiac patient, both within hospital and after discharge. The material making up the book has therefore, wherever possible, been presented in a nondisciplinary way; the intention has been to advance the view that sensitivity to the cardiac patient's behavioral and psychological needs is the responsibility not only of those trained in psychology but of all those involved in the management of the patient. It is hoped, in this respect, that the book will add a greater clinical awareness among all those involved with medical management. Nonetheless, it is most likely that the actual responsibility for the psychological care and behavioral management of the cardiac patient will fall to the clinical psychologist or someone similarly trained. In view of this, the book has been given a very deliberate structure that seeks to acquaint the nonmedically trained practitioner with the anatomy, pathology, and epidemiology of coronary heart disease before progressing to a consideration, more central to the text, of the actual procedures of psychological and behavioral management.

The first chapter is necessarily a derivative one presenting concrete biological information and accepting this to be a statement of undisputed fact. As such, the material contained in it may be found, in similar form, in any of a large number of medical texts. In the case of information so enshrined in medical wisdom, it is difficult to find any departure from a standard line, however where issues have been less than totally clear, I have relied on the authority of two recent and excellent volumes on cardiology. These are Willerson and Sanders's edited work

Clinical Cardiology with its many valuable contributions, and Willerson, Hillis, and Buja's encyclopedic text *Ischemic Heart Disease*. Where these two volumes have been drawn on, they have been appropriately cited in the text, and if the citation of their contents is frequent, it is a tribute to their clarity. I have also drawn on the National Cooperative Pooling Project data to illustrate points of cardiovascular epidemiology in the latter part of the first chapter, since these data present the most clear-cut demonstrations of the role of risk factors in the determination of coronary heart disease.

Material for the remaining chapters has been derived largely from work published in the past decade or so in appropriate psychological and medical journals. Two comments may be made on this process. Firstly, while one tries to be exhaustive in the process of the collection of material, using all possible bibliographic and referencing sources, a small amount of material that some might consider important will invariably fail to emerge from the search. The writing of each chapter of the book was preceded by a computer search of the literature, though the fallibility of this procedure, slight as it is, must be admitted. For those whose work was not cited and who believe this to be a major omission, I can only agree. Secondly, while one tries to be completely dispassionate in reviewing published material, drawing conclusions from it and organizing it into the structure of a chapter, one must inevitably make judgments both on the merits of a particular area and on the implications which any area has for clinical practice. Responsibility for these judgments is mine alone. They were made with all possible objectivity and in the light of experience, and while some may wish to argue the emphasis of the evidence in other ways, this is of course the essence of scientific debate.

I am indebted to a number of people, directly or indirectly, for the work leading to the production of this book. Emeritus Professor Malcolm Whyte first introduced me to the psychological study of coronary heart disease and I will always highly value his collaboration in a number of studies. On a number of occasions, I have had the privilege of working with Dr. Ray Rosenman and I am grateful to have been given the benefit of his wisdom and intellect. The patience of the Ablex Publishing Corporation and the continued faith of the editor of this series on clinical psychology, Dr. Glenn Caddy, have done much to soothe the anxiety associated with the production of a book. My thanks must also go to Mrs. Jess Giddings and her staff of secretaries in the Department of Psychology at the Australian National University for their expert and patient typing of the several drafts of the manuscript. Finally, it is a pleasure to acknowledge the help of my wife, Dr. Anne Foon, who, despite her own workload, read every chapter, corrected my spelling, commented on my expression, offered advice (always taken up) on content, and confirmed yet again her inestimable worth.

D.G.B.
Canberra, 1985

CHAPTER 1

The Pathology and Epidemiology of Coronary Heart Disease

1. THE ANATOMY OF THE HEART AND CIRCULATION

1.1 Gross Anatomy

The human heart is a four-chambered organ the sole purpose of which is to provide the pumping force necessary for the circulation of the blood to the body. It sits in the left thoracic cavity and is oriented such that its apex lies immediately posterior to the sternum at around the level of the fifth intercostal space. A plane defined by the interatrial and interventricular septa forms an angle of between 40° and 45°, with a vertical plane bisecting the sternum and vertebral column.

The heart is fixed within the thoracic cavity by means of the pericardial sac. This sac, composed of layers of collagen tissue, fits closely around the epicardial surface of the heart and is separated from the heart by pericardial fluid. This fluid serves a lubricating function, since the human heart is in constant motion. The pericardial sac in turn is attached at various points, both to the diaphragm and to the sternum by a series of ligaments.

The tissue of the heart is composed of a series of muscle layers, the nature and disposition of which are concisely described by Caufield (1977). The musculature of the heart, which can be collectively termed the myocardium, is formed during embryological development into four precisely interconnected chambers. The atria, which are situated in the superior (upper) part of the heart, are separated from the ventricles, which are situated in the inferior (lower) part of the heart, by a fibrous ring of muscle bundles. Both the atria and ventricles are divided into right and left sections by septa. The flow of blood between the various chambers of the heart is, in the healthy individual, quite strictly regulated by the presence of valves.

Venous blood enters the right atrium by means of the superior vena cava and descends through the tricuspid valve into the right ventricle. At a point where the myocardium is relaxed (diastole), this flow is unimpaired, however, when the myocardium is in a state of contraction (systole), the tricuspid valve closes to prevent the backflow of blood into the right atrium. During systole, blood is pumped from the right ventricle through the pulmonary arteries to the lungs where a process of gas exchange takes place and venous blood becomes reoxygenated by hemoglobin uptake of oxygen to form arterial blood. This blood is returned to the left atrium by means of the pulmonary veins. It descends through the mitral valve into the left ventricle and finally, during systole, is ejected through the ascending aorta into the circulatory system to supply the organs of the body. Backflow of blood from the left ventricle to the left atrium during systole is prevented by the closure of the mitral valve. Similarly, backflow of blood from the large aortic vessel into the left ventricle during diastole is prevented by the closure of the aortic valve. Filling of the ventricles with blood occurs largely during ventricular diastole, though this is enhanced by atrial contraction. Pressure within the ventricles is somewhat higher than that within the atria and impairment of valve function allowing the backflow of blood from ventricles to atria places considerable strain upon the heart. This is most often seen in mitral-valve incompetence.

The rhythm of systole and diastole which is necessary for the maintenance of an adequate blood supply to the body is regulated by a series of motor fibers arising from the autonomic nervous system and embedded at various points in the myocardium. Both sympathetic and parasympathetic fibers are represented in this system and neurophysiological disruptions may have serious ramifications for the efficient functioning of the heart. The system is made more sophisticated by the presence of pressure receptors (baro-receptors) within the major arteries that feed back information related to blood pressure and can act to modify cardiac output.

Both the degree and efficiency of blood flow to the body are, however, a complex function of a number of attributes including heart rate, blood pressure, the ejection fraction (the volume of blood ejected from the left ventricle during systole), the resistance of the circulatory system within the various body organs to the flow of blood (Surwit, Williams, & Shapiro, 1982). While a detailed consideration of the neurophysiological and hemodynamic factors regulating the circulation of blood is beyond the scope of this book, a number of recent accounts (Braunwald, Ross, & Sonnenblick, 1976; Surwit et al., 1982) will provide a more than adequate grounding in this area. Needless to say, any impairment to the integrity of the myocardium, which is the central theme of this book, will have serious implications for the efficient delivery of blood through the circulatory system to the organs of the body.

1.2   The Coronary Arteries

The heart, in conjunction with arteries conveying blood from it and veins returning blood to it, forms a closed circulatory system within the body. As Surwit et al. (1982) have remarked, the central purpose of this system is to meet the metabolic needs of the body by way of the delivery of oxygen and nutrient substances to body tissues and the removal of body wastes. As a functional organ in its own right, however, the heart has fundamental metabolic needs that must also be supplied by the circulation of blood within the myocardium. This circulation is undertaken by the coronary arteries.

The precise anatomy of the coronary circulation varies from one individual to another, though the basis for this is formed by two arteries—the right coronary artery, which arises from the right aortic sinus, and the left common coronary artery, which arises from the left aortic sinus. Circulation to the myocardium surrounding the right ventricle is undertaken by the right coronary artery and brances arising from it, though the precise course of this arterial system is both complex and variable. The left common coronary artery branches into the left anterior descending artery and the left circumflex artery, which together circulate blood to the left side of the myocardium and in particular to the tissue surrounding the left ventricle. As the coronary arteries branch into progressively smaller vessels, so as to serve broader areas of the myocardium, a detailed network of arterioles and capillaries can be seen ultimately to supply blood to individual muscle cells. Deoxygenated blood is taken up by the coronary veins which form parallel though reverse networks to the arterial system. The bulk of the deoxygenated blood from the coronary circulation enters the right atrium and rejoins the systemic process.

The cellular structure of the coronary arteries has been the topic of whole volumes and need not be dwelt upon here. It is important, however, to touch briefly on the structure of the internal surface of the coronary arteries as damage to this structure forms the basis of cornary-artery disease and finally of coronary heart disease.

The epicardial coronary arteries are essentially elastic in form and are therefore fitted to accommodate cardiac output at relatively high pressures during ventricular contraction and to revert to low-pressure conduction systems during diastole. The physical properties of this elasticity in relation to the coronary circulation have been discussed in detail by Caulfield (1977). The internal lining of the coronary arteries consists of endothelial cells that are tightly bound to a basement membrane. This is in turn attached to the underlying stroma by filaments of collagen. The endothelial surface of the coronary arteries is normally smooth and allows for the unhindered passage of blood. However, when damage occurs to the endothelial cell lining there are several immediate pathological consequences. The first is that the flow of blood within the bloodstream becomes disturbed. Secondly, the damaged lining of the vessel wall forms a focus for the deposit of dissolved foreign matter precipitating out of the bloodstream. This in turn lays the foundation for the formation of atherosclerotic deposits which, if progressive, may finally result in the occlusion of the coronary arteries. Finally, since tissue containing collagen is thrombogenic, its exposure to blood increases the possibility of the formation of blood clots and thus also of blockage within the coronary arteries.

Disease of the coronary arteries, however this comes about, forms the substrate for clinical coronary heart disease. The maintenance of healthy coronary arteries is perhaps the single-most-important step in the prevention of coronary heart disease. A wide range of factors bear on the production of cornary-artery disease and an equally wide range of factors join with coronary-artery disease to precipitate clinical episodes of cornary heart disease. Perhaps the most central issue relevant to the former, however, is that of atherosclerosis.

2.   PATHOLOGICAL AND CLINICAL CONSIDERATIONS

2.1   Atherosclerosis

Flaherty and Weisfeldt (1977) in a recent discussion of coronary heart disease stated that in the overwhelming majority of cases this is the "end result of the pathologic process designated as coronary atherosclerosis." While a number of other causes have been postulated and in particular the sudden and largely unexplained spasm of coronary arteries, the bulk of opinion continues to lie with atherosclerotic damage to the coronary arteries as the most central precursor of coronary heart disease.

The basis of coronary atherosclerosis in turn is atheroma or atherosclerotic plaque. Pathological changes associated with this process involve the deposition of fatty substances, carried by blood, into the internal cellular structure of the coronary artery wall. It is possible that damage to the microstructure of the coronary-artery wall provides a focus for this deposit, though the mechanisms leading to such damage are complex. This progressive pathology ultimately proliferates and destroys the internal surface of the elastic coronary arteries, the process being accompanied by fibrosis and calcification so that the end result is both thickening and hardening of the arterial walls. At the very least the consequences of the atherosclerotic process are a reduction in blood supply to parts of the myocardium distal to the arterial narrowing and local turbulence of the blood flow at points around the arterial lesion. However, in a significant proportion of persons with severe atherosclerotic damage the aggregation of blood platelets, under the influence of a variety of thrombogenic factors, can lead to the formation of a thrombus or blood clot at one or other points in the coronary artery and hence to the complete occlusion of that vessel. The most obvious result of this is a complete cessation of blood supply to points in the myocardium further on from the blockage and the very rapid death or necrosis of myocardial tissue denied its regular blood supply. Necrosis of the myocardium can occur within two minutes of the cessation of blood flow.

2.2   Coronary Heart Disease

The clinical signs of coronary-artery occlusion are several. Dimunition of blood supply to points in the myocardium will eventually result in a myocardial demand for oxygen that is unable to be met by the reduced blood volume able to be transported through diseased coronary arteries. The most immediate result of this is the condition of myocardial ischemia, whereby the myocardium, starved of an adequate blood supply, builds up lactic acid and other toxic waste products within muscle tissue. The clinical consequence of this disruption to myocardial metabolism is that of ischemic pain, which is clinically termed angina pectoris. This may occur either spontaneously or duing physical exertion, when the demand by the myocardium for oxygen is markedly in excess of its normal requirements. However, in some patients with quite severe disease of the coronary arteries, angina pectoris can be experienced even during times of bed rest. Coincident with this clinical condition is a greater or lesser decrease in the efficiency of the heart to maintain bodily circulation and, therefore, a variety of clinical symptoms ranging from tiredness and breathlessness to an almost complete incapacity to undertake physical work, these symptoms being in rough proportion to the extent of disease within the coronary arteries.

The increasing sophistication of medical investigatory techniques, and principally the use of coronary angiographic procedures, has allowed the early diagnosis of coronary-artery disease before the patient experiences ischemic symptoms or discomfort of any severe kind. Increasingly often such patients are referred for coronary-bypass surgery, where a piece of healthy blood vessel usually taken from the same individual is grafted so as to shunt blood around a diseased portion of a coronary artery and restore circulation to the associated myocardial tissue. This process is sometimes aided by the natural growth of collateral vessels to compensate for the deficiencies of the diseased artery. However, a sizable number of patients with symptoms of angina, usually secondary to quite severe disease of the coronary arteries, go on to experience one or more episodes of coronary heart disease.

Though the precise mechanisms underlying complete coronary occlusion are still not totally understood, it is clear that severe narrowing of the coronary arteries in conjunction with the presence of conditions that facilitate clotting of the blood may result in the aggregation of blood platelets and the formation of a blood clot that totally occludes the coronary artery. The subsequent cessation of blood supply results in very rapid death of myocardial tissue distal to the point of occlusion and this loss of myocardial tissue is clinically termed myocardial infarction. Once lost, this tissue is not regeneratable and while other areas of the myocardium may be strengthened by physical exercise and while collateral circulation from other coronary arteries to surrounding areas of the myocardium may be established to maintain blood supply to intact muscle tissue, the total integrity of the myocardium and its subsequent efficiency in accomplishing an adequate systemic circulation has been decreased to an extent related to the amount of tissue loss.

Another potential mechanism more recently implicated in the precipitation of coronary occlusion has been that of coronary-artery vasospasm. While the processes underlying this are less clearly understood than those forming the basis of coronary thrombosis, the most likely determinant would appear to be an acute discharge of sympathetic neurones both in and of the coronary-artery wall, resulting in a total but transient constriction of the vessel and a cessation of blood flowing through it. Thus while the vasospasm may subside and the coronary artery reopen to re-establish blood supply to the myocardium, the result is nonetheless an area of myocardial necrosis and, therefore, of myocardial infarction. This mechanism has been linked particularly to the syndrome of sudden cardiac death, where postmortem examinations of patients who have died suddenly have revealed substantial areas of myocardial necrosis in the absence of significant coronary-artery disease (Steptoe, 1981).

However, whatever the mechanisms underlying coronary-artery occlusion, the clinical symptoms associated with acute myocardial infarction are usually quite characteristic. These consist of severe retrosternal pain, usually described as constricting in nature and similar to anginal pain, together with nausea, faintness, loss of breath, and palpitations. In some cases the patient may lose consciousness. This pain may radiate to the left arm and, less commonly, to the throat and angles of the jaw. On clinical examination the patient is occasionally white and sweating with an irregular pulse due to extra systolic beats. In a set of formal guidelines on the diagnosis of coronary heart disease for research purposes, the World Health Organization (1973) listed the following history of chest pain as that most typically signaling the onset of myocardial infarction. In the usual case, pain is (a) diffused through the chest either anteriorly or generally, though it may remain localized in the chest or radiate to the shoulder, arms, jaws, or abdomen on one or both sides; (b) resistant to nitroglycerine; (c) of a duration of more than 20 minutes; and (d) of severe or agonizing intensity. An atypical history is more likely to include symptoms such as dyspnea, a feeling of suffocation, "indigestion," syncope, general malaise, sweating, or acute cardiac failure. Blood pressure is frequently elevated during the first few hours, though it often decreases to normal levels after this. In some cases both coldness and cyanosis of the extremities may be seen, both of which indicate a disturbance in the efficiency of the circulatory system.

A number of clinical conditions, including infections of the pericardium, may mimic some symptoms of myocardial infarction, and particularly those of chest pain. Diagnosis of myocardial infarction is, therefore, dependent on a series of electrophysiological and laboratory investigations in the first days following the onset of symptoms. Characteristic electrocardiographic (EKG) changes are found in over 95% of patients shortly after the onset of chest pain (Fleming & Brainbridge, 1967). In order to attract an unequivocal diagnosis of myocardial infarction, the World Health Organization (1973) has determined that these should involve (a) the development of a pathological Q wave, and (b) the evolution of an injury current lasting for more than one day. (This necessitates the collection of serial EKG traces in order to confirm these changes over a period of time.) The World Health Organization's guidelines go on to indicate a series of EKG changes providing more equivocal evidence of myocardial infarction, including (a) the presence of an injury current which later disappears, (b) the presence of a stationary injury current, (c) symmetrical inversions of the T wave, (d) bundle-branch block with additional Q wave, and (e) presence of a pathological Q wave in a single EKG record.

In addition to clinical history of chest pain and the detection of EKG changes, it is also necessary to establish the presence in the blood of certain enzymes indicating the process of myocardial tissue necrosis. Typically, this process results in the presence of serum glutamic oxaloacetic transaminase (SGOT) and lactic dehydrogenase (LDH), the former appearing in elevated levels between eight and 36 hours after myocardial infarction and the latter peaking at between three and six days after the clinical event (Willerson, Hillis, & Buja, 1982). The presence of all three of these signs provides almost certain evidence of myocardial infarction.

3. RISK FACTORS FOR CORONARY HEART DISEASE

It should be clear, even from this brief review of the pathological processes underlying coronary heart disease, that these mechanisms are complex and still not completely understood. Epidemiological studies employing large samples of subjects have, however, established statistical associations of varying degrees between a variety of factors and the risk of sustaining either coronary-artery disease or myocardial infarction. While there is considerable debate as to the relative importance of these risk factors and even more debate as to the mechanisms through which they exert their influence on the coronary arterial system, an overview of the nature and potency of the more consistently indicated of these risk factors would appear germane to the substance of this book. Willerson et al. (1982) provide a useful and comprehensive list of risk factors for the development of coronary heart disease. These are conveniently divided into the categories of risk factors related to fundamental biology (e.g., age, sex, and inherited characteristics), those related to endogenous regulatory mechanisms (e.g., hypertension, hyperlipidemia, and the relative ratios of blood-fat fractions), those concerned with environmental factors (e.g., cigarette smoking, physical activity, and psychological and behavioral characteristics) and those to do with organ-system pathology (e.g., chronic renal disease or hypothyroidism). The bulk of epidemiological evidence, however, indicates that four risk factors, namely high serum lipids, high blood pressure, cigarette smoking, and presence of a characteristic pattern of time-pressured, hard-driven, and sometimes aggressive behaviors (the Type A behavior pattern), contribute most strongly and most consistently to risk of coronary heart disease.

3.1   Serum Lipids

The evidence documenting associations between elevated levels of serum lipids and the incidence of coronary heart disease is both large and variable. The association achieved strong and popular recognition with a study of Keys (1970) showing that population rates of coronary heart disease were positively correlated with population levels of serum cholesterol. This was closely followed by the publication of data from the National Cooperative Pooling Project in the U.S.A. (Doyle & Kannel, 1970) showing rates of first major coronary events as 45 per 1,000 in men with serum-cholesterol levels of 175 mg % rising to rates of 162 per 1,000 in men with serum-cholesterol rates greater than 300 mg %. These data are summarised in Fig. 1.1 below.

Data in general agreement with this trend have been reported by Stamler (1974), Kannel, McGee, and Gordon (1976) and Rosenman, Brand, Jenkins, Friedman, Straus, and Wurm (1975). Based on data such as these, it would seem that approximately one-third of survivors of acute myocardial infarction aged 60 years or less are characterized by an elevation of lipids in the blood (Willerson et al., 1982).

While this evidence is both persuasive and has become enshrined in conventional medical wisdom, a number of questions remain to be answered. The first

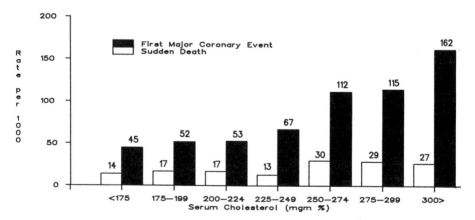

Figure 1.1   National Cooperative Pooling Project—Serum cholesterol at entry and 10-year age-adjusted rates per 1,000 men for first major coronary event, including fatal or survived myocardial infarctions or sudden death only from heart disease (redrawn from Circulation, Vol. 42, 1970).

concerns the mechanisms responsible for the regulation of serum lipid levels. Biosynthesis of cholesterol, which appears to be the lipid substance most implicated in the pathology of coronary artery disease (the role of triglycerides as an independent risk factor is very much more contentious), occurs primarily in the liver (Willerson et al., 1982). Cholesterol attaches to protein molecules of varying densities and is thereby transported to peripheral tissues. The biochemistry of this process has been extensively investigated (Gotto, Miller, & Oliver, 1978; Schaefer, Eisenberg, & Levy, 1978), and while the issue is indeed a complex one, it is not by and large controversial. Cholesterol attached to low-density lipoprotein (LDL) is strongly associated with the risk of coronary heart disease while levels of high-density lipoprotein (HDL) appear to have a consistently negative association with coronary-heart-disease risk.

What is controversial is the role of diet in the regulation of serum lipids. While Keys's (1970) study popularized the notion that diet, insofar as it influences serum lipids, can be a coronary risk factor, and while this has more recently attracted some epidemiological support (Shekelle, Shryock, Paul, Lepper, Stamler, Liu, & Raynor, 1981) there is now evidence at odds with this opinion (Byrne, Rosenman, & Schiller, 1985). Questioning of the evidence linking diet, serum cholesterol and coronary heart disease has arisen both from methodological concerns (Armstrong, Mann, Adelstein, & Eskin, 1975; Mann, 1977) and because of conflicting epidemiological data (Nichols, Ravenscroft, Lamphiear, & Ostrander, 1976; Byrne et al., 1985). Findings failing to relate diet to serum cholesterol have cast doubt on the area and while the association between serum cholesterol and risk of coronary heart disease must continue to be given credence, the regulation of this risk factor by means of patterns of dietary intake is indeed contentious; one must look to a very much more complex set of determinants in order to explain levels of cholesterol in the blood. The role of behavior in the regulation of serum lipids has attracted particular attention recently (Dimsdale & Heid, 1982) and the environment-person interaction presents itself as a fertile area for future epidemiological study of the risk of coronary heart disease endowed by serum lipids.

3.2   Blood Pressure

Once more, data from the National Cooperative Pooling Project (1970, 1978) can be used to demonstrate the role of blood pressure as a coronary risk factor. These data show that men with a diastolic pressure of less than 75 mm Hg have an age-adjusted rate of first major coronary events of 48 per 1,000, whereas men with diastolic pressure of 105 mm Hg or greater, have an age-adjusted risk rate for major coronary events of 188 per 1,000. This risk pattern can best be seen in Fig. 1.2 below. The World Health Organization considers the area of risk to include diastolic pressures of 95 mm Hg and greater and in the range of 95-104 mm Hg the age-adjusted rate for first major coronary events was 99 per 1,000. It

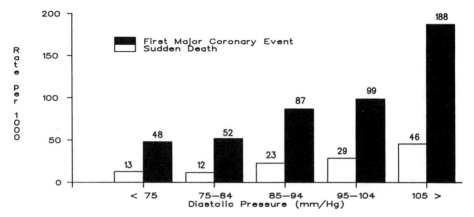

Figure 1.2   National Cooperative Project—Diastolic blood pressure at entry and 10-year age-adjusted rates per 1,000 men for first major coronary event, including fatal or survived myocardial infarctions or sudden death only from heart disease (redrawn from Circulation, Vol. 42, 1970).

is quite clear from these data that increases in diastolic pressure constitute a noticeable risk for coronary heart disease.

A similar picture is evident for systolic blood pressure. Data from the National Cooperative Pooling Project (1970, 1978) show a steady rise in the incidence of both sudden cardiac death and first major survived coronary events in middle-aged men in parallel with increases in systolic blood pressure. Thus, while the psychophysiological mechanisms underlying the determination of blood pressure are complex and continue to be subject to intensive investigation (Steptoe, 1981; Surwit et al., 1982), high blood pressure is a risk factor for coronary heart disease which must continue to be accorded serious concern.

3.3   Cigarette Smoking

Data from a variety of sources continue to confirm the association between cigarette smoking and risk of coronary heart disease. The National Cooperative Pooling Project (1970, 1978) reported the death rate from coronary heart disease to be 20 per 1,000 from men who have never smoked in contrast to a death rate of 60 per 1,000 among men who had smoked greater than one packet of cigarettes per week. This death rate fell in proportion to decreases in the number of cigarettes smoked per day. Moreover, it was shown that while pipe and cigar smoking introduced a modest increase in risk of death from coronary heart disease, it was not substantially above that for nonsmokers and was certainly considerably below that for cigarette smokers. This may have something to do with differential rates of absorption of toxic substances from cigarette smoking in the lungs and in the buccal cavity; cigarette smokers tend to inhale into the lungs whereas cigar and pipe smokers are more likely to keep the smoke within the mouth. The evidence here, however, is somewhat tenuous. Most interestingly, the rate of coronary-heart-disease deaths among those who had smoked in the past but had subsequently given up was marginally below the coronary-heart-disease death rate for those who had never smoked. These rates are represented in Fig. 1.3.

Reported risk attributed to cigarette smoking was rather greater when the first major survived coronary event and not coronary-heart-disease death consituted the epidemiological end point. In this case the risk associated with past smoking was greater than that associated with those who had never smoked cigarettes. In all other respects however the pattern of risk for survived coronary heart disease among smokers paralleled that found for coronary-heart-disease deaths.

More recently, a succession of reports from the United States Surgeon General (see for example United States Surgeon General's report on smoking and health, 1979) have consistently reported strong epidemiological associations between cigarette smoking and risk of coronary heart disease. The Surgeon General's report for 1979 cited 26 major epidemiological studies in which it was shown that smokers had a higher incidence of heart attacks, both fatal and nonfatal, than did nonsmokers. Particularly impressive among this evidence are the results from the American Cancer Society study. It involved a large cohort of men and women between ages 40 and 79. Follow-up rate over six years was 99%, and this yielded a final sample of 358,534 men and 445,875 women, of whom 10,771

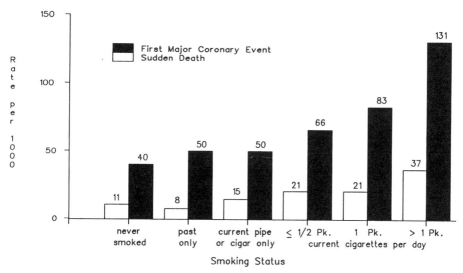

Figure 1.3   National Cooperative Pooling Project—Smoking status at entry and 10-year age adjusted rates per 1,000 men for first major coronary event, including fatal or survived myocardial infarctions or sudden death only from heart disease (redrawn from *Circulation*, Vol. 42, 1970).

men and 4,048 women had died of an episode of coronary heart disease at some stage during the follow-up period. While risk of death from coronary heart disease clearly varied with age, there was a significant excess of coronary-heart-disease deaths among smokers relative to nonsmokers. This held for both men and women and for all age groups (Hammond & Garfinkel, 1969).

While the mechanisms linking cigarette smoking with damage to coronary arteries and to initiation of coronary heart disease are somewhat poorly understood, there is evidence that these links might act both through the exacerbation of existing coronary-artery atherosclerosis and also by the production of regional cardiac ischemia, which in turn may promote electrical instability, fibrillation, and ultimate destabilization of electrical conduction within the myocardium. On the basis of evidence such as this it can be concluded that cigarette smoking constitutes one of the strongest risks for coronary heart disease (Donovan & Hodge, 1980).

3.4   Type A Behavior

Among all risk factors for coronary heart disease, this is the newest and perhaps most controversial. The issue of Type A behavior is sufficiently important to the theme of this book for its definitions and descriptions to be dealt with in detail (see Chapter 8). Briefly, however, the Type A Behavior Pattern is characterized by a sense of time urgency, a high need for achievement and excessive ambition, impatience and intolerance of frustration, an unusual degree of job involvement, and overt hostility and aggression (Byrne, 1981). While Type A behavior has been linked with the incidence of coronary heart disease in a number of retrospective and prospective studies, three of these studies stand out for their magnitude and rigor.

The Western Collaborative Group Study (Rosenman et al., 1975) assessed Type A behavior in 3,154 male subjects who were healthy at the time of initial examination. These subjects were followed through for 8.5 years during which serial medical examinations and other investigations provided close to complete data on coronary events, whether survived or otherwise. Simultaneous adjustment for all other risk factors at termination of the study revealed that Type A men had had between 1.87 and 1.98 times more risk of coronary heart disease over 8.5 years than did men in whom Type A behavior was not evident.

Similar results emerged from an eight-year follow-up of subjects in Framingham Study (Haynes, Feinleib, & Kannel, 1980). Taking all other risk factors into account, male subjects between 45 and 54 years of age who had Type A behavior showed a risk of coronary heart disease around 50% greater than men in the same age group who were not Type A. When men between 55 and 64 years were considered, the risk of coronary heart disease attributable to Type A behavior increased to twice that relative to men without the behavior pattern.

In a major retrospective study involving more than 6,000 employees in Belgian industrial organizations, the presence of Type A behavior was also found to be strongly related to the prevalence of identified coronary heart disease; this was independent of other coronary risk factors (Kornitzer, Kittel, DeBacker, & Dramaix, 1981).

A number of issues remain to be resolved regarding Type A behavior as a coronary risk. A great deal of work remains to be done both on the definition and measurement of Type A behavior (Byrne, Rosenman, Chesney & Schiller, 1985). Moreover, the pathophysiological links between the Type A behavior pattern and coronary-artery pathology are yet to be established with any certainty. Still, the weight of evidence from well-conducted epidemiological studies clearly indicates the Type A behavior pattern as an independent and causal risk factor for coronary heart disease.

3.5   The Additivity of Coronary Risk Factors

The discussion to this point has concerned the potency of single risk factors considered independently of all other risk factors. While it is of course possible for an individual to have only one of a number of coronary risk factors, it is more likely the case that a single individual will possess several risk factors in combination. The rules by which these risk factors add together are not well understood and are almost certainly a function of the relative level of risk factors in any individual. Nonetheless, there are some data from major epidemiological studies dealing with the additivity at least of the three risk factors of serum cholesterol, high blood pressure, and cigarette smoking.

This situation, too, can be represented by data from the National Cooperative Pooling Project (1970) that can be seen in Fig. 1.4 below. The age-adjusted rate for a first major coronary event (myocardial infarction) among cigarette smokers with normal blood pressure and serum cholesterol levels is somewhat more than twice that for persons with no risk factors. The presence of high blood pressure or serum cholesterol, again in the absence of other risk factors, raises the rate of first major coronary events marginally higher even than this. A combination of any two risk factors raises the rate of illness events to between three and four times that where no risk factors are in evidence, while the presence of all three risk factors (high blood pressure, elevated serum cholesterol, and cigarette smoking) almost doubles the rate of first major coronary events relative to the effects of two risk factors only.

There is no precise formula that can explain the ways in which coronary risk factors combine to increase the observed rates of myocardial infarction. It is unlikely to involve a simple process of addition since each risk factor would not appear to carry equal weight in the determination of risk. On the other hand, the data from the National Cooperative Pooling Project (1970, 1978) as well as

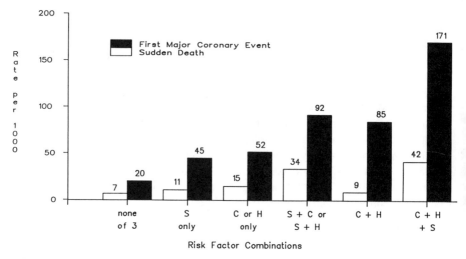

Figure 1.4 National Cooperative Pooling Project—Combinations of three risk factors (S—smoking, C—elevated cholesterol, H—hypertension) at entry and age-adjusted rates per 1,000 men for first major coronary event, including fatal or survived myocardial infarctions or sudden death only from heart disease (redrawn from Circulation, Vol. 42, 1970).

evidence from a persuasive body of independent epidemiological studies accumulating over the past two decades indicates quite conclusively that high blood pressure, elevated levels of cholesterol (and perhaps other lipid substances) in the blood, and cigarette smoking, either singly or in combination, endow substantially increased risks of sustaining coronary heart disease.

4. THE DISTRIBUTION OF CORONARY HEART DISEASE

4.1 Rates of Coronary Heart Disease

It should be clear from the preceding section that rates of coronary heart disease in the community at large are determined by a range of factors, not the least of which are community levels of the various risk factors. Thus, for example, coronary heart disease is more apparent in communities where dietary cholesterol intake or cigarett-smoking levels are high than in communities where these risk factors are less in evidence (Armstrong, Mann, Adelstein, & Eskin, 1975). Both age and sex are also strongly and characteristically related to rates of coronary heart disease. By and large, the risk of myocardial infarction increases with age in a roughly linear fashion (Pole, McCall, Reader, & Woodings, 1977), while at least for those under 60 years of age, women show a substantially lower rate of coronary heart disease than men (Johnson, 1977).

Both age and sex differentials in coronary heart disease are well illustrated by recent data on attack and case fatality rates for acute myocadial infarction over a one-year period within a single community representing a broad range of social and occupational strata (Leeder, Dobson, Gibberd, & Flynn, 1983). These data were collected in accordance with the methodological guidelines laid down by the World Health Organization for the collection of data on the incidence of myocardial infarction, and are, therefore, comparable with data from many other studies of the incidence of myocardial infarction both in Europe and North America. The study population consisted of 238,028 men and women aged 20 to 69 years and rates of myocardial infarction were expressed in terms of numbers/1,000/year. In this sample, myocardial infarction was nonexistent in both men and women under the age of 25, and rates were very small up to the age of 39. Indeed, cumulative rates for all subjects to 39 years for both definite and possible acute myocardial infarction were only 4.1/1,000/year for men and 0.7/1,000/year for women. By contast, for the age group 65 to 69 years, the rates rose to 42.4/1,000/year for men and 20.7/1,000/year for women. This increase with age of between 10 and 20 fold is characteristic of the relationship to be seen between age and coronary heart disease. To the degree that coronary heart disease involves the progressive development of coronary atherosclerosis, it is perhaps not surprising that the illness event serving as the epidemiological end point should bear a strong relationship to age. The sex differentials also apparent from the data are rather less easy to explain.

It can be seen that in the earlier age groups, men are more likely than women, by a ratio of about six to one, to sustain an acute myocardial infarction. Though this discrepancy in rates evens up somewhat in later years, the ratio of coronary events in men relative to women remains at around two to one even in the 65-to 69-year age group. Johnson (1977) was unable to explain this sex difference in terms of consistent differences in levels of the most prominent risk factors for coronary heart disease, finding instead that women maintain lower rates of myocardial infarction despite, in some instances, relatively higher levels of risk factors.

Though the data are somewhat more sparse, socio-occupational influences on rates of myocardial infarction have also been reported. A large British study using a cohort of 17,530 civil servants (Marmot, Rose, Shipley, & Hamilton, 1978) found that men in the lowest grades of employment had around 3.6 times the mortality from coronary heart disease than did men in higher grades of employment in the British Civil Service. In this instance, too, there was no satisfactory explanation in terms of difference in levels of the major risk factors.

Cross-cultural variation in rates of coronary heart disease is now sufficiently well documented to add to the overall epidemiological picture. Data from the

National Heart and Lung Institute (1971), which can be seen in Fig. 1.5 here show a gradient in yearly incidence rates across a selection of developed countries, ranging from almost 500/100,000 in Finland, through around 370/100,000 in the United States and Australia, down to less than 100/100,000 in Japan. While some of this can almost certainly be explained by variation in the levels of the standard risk factors for coronary heart disease, the structure and characteristics of the culture itself must be taken into account.

This contribution is perhaps made most evident by the work of Marmot and Syme (1976) in a study of acculturation and coronary heart disease in Japanese-Americans. Several research reports have documented a gradient in rates of coronary heart disease across Japanese living in Japan, those living in Hawaii, and those living in the United States, with lowest rates occurring among the first of these groups and highest rates among the last. This difference could not be explained in terms of a parallel gradient in the levels of standard risk factors. By way of confirmation, Marmot and Syme (1976) examined a sample of 3,809

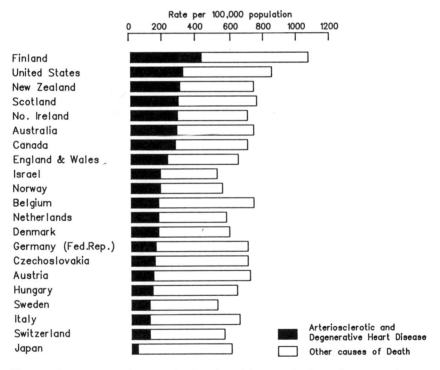

Figure 1.5   Death rates from arteriosclerotic and degenerative heart disease and from all causes; selected countries, 1967–men aged 45–54 years (redrawn from Arteriosclerosis, Vol. 1, 1971).

persons of Japanese ancestry living in the United States and graded according to the degree to which they held to traditional Japanese cultural values. Once more, it was found that those holding most closely to the Japanese culture had lower rates of coronary heart disease than those adopting North American cultural styles. Moreover, this gradient, too, was found to be largely independent of the prevailing levels of standard risk factors, thus recommending an interpretation phrased in terms of behavioral and social considerations.

4.2 The Scope of the Problem

In view of the variation in rates of coronary heart disease by age, sex, occupation, culture, and perhaps other variables, it is not a simple matter to express community levels in terms of a single numerical index. The National Heart and Lung Institute in the United States reported (1971) that in 1967 approximately one million deaths (representing 54% of the yearly death rate for that country) could be attributed to diseases of the cardiovascular system.

The establishment of myocardial infarction registers in several centers in Europe, North America, and the Pacific region, partly under the aegis of the World Health Organization, has allowed the collection of more precise data on the incidence of the disease and on its clinical course. The hallmark of this work has been the attention to methodological detail both with respect to the accuracy of diagnosis and completeness of the samples, and a small but representative overview of several major studies will serve to illustrate the extent of coronary heart disease within Western, developed societies.

Each study cited considers incidence data for acute myocardial infarction within a well-defined population over a single year. While rates clearly vary according to age, mean figures only will be referred to, though of course rates will tend to fall below the mean for younger groups of patients and above it for those in older age groups. The Framinham Study of coronary-heart-disease risk is often considered to be the benchmark in the epidemiological investigation of the cardiovascular diseases. The one-year incidence of first acute myocardial infarction in this Northeastern United States community was around 657/100,000 for men and 117/100,000 for women all aged between 35 and 64 years (Kannel, Dawber, & McNamara, 1966). In a somewhat more industrialized part of the United States, marginally lower rates of 613/100,000 for men and 110/100,000 for women of the same age group were reported (Pell & D'Alonzo, 1963). Data from the Norwegian city of Oslo revealed somewhat lower rates of 572/100,000 for men but comparable rates of 115/100,000 for women (Westlund, 1965), while in the Perth region of Australia, rates of first acute myocardial infarction were 554/100,000 for men and 173/100,000 for women, this time in the age range of 30 to 69 years (Pole, McCall, Reader, & Woodings, 1977). These rates rose to 740/100,000 for men and 220/100,000 for women when all (first or subsequent) coronary events were considered, and were much in accord with data reported for a geographically separate region on the east coast of Australia (Leeder et al., 1983). While the rates for coronary heart disease in Australia were similar to those of North America and Europe for men, rates among Australian women were somewhat in excess of those evident in the Northern Hemisphere.

While rates of coronary heart disease will clearly vary according to communities, circumstances and the characteristics of population, these data should give a good indication of the degree to which Western societies are troubled by the disease. There is some evidence of movement in rates over past years, with coronary-heart-disease mortality decreasing in some countries (notably Belgium, Finland, Norway, the United States, Canada, and Australia) but remaining stable in many others (World Health Organization, 1981). The reason for this movement is not to be found in variations in levels of standard risk factors. Moreover, the data are for coronary mortality only, and may not reflect overall levels of survived myocardial infarction. This aside, the preceding brief overview can do nothing but reinforce the now often-heard claim that coronary heart disease in Western societies remains in epidemic proportions.

CHAPTER 2

Outcomes After Myocardial Infarction

1. THE CONSEQUENCES OF MYOCARDIAL INFARCTION

Myocardial infarction is a life-threatening illness. Its occurrence carries twin risks for the future. The first is death; the second is continued and lengthy disability, both physical and psychological. The management of the patient with myocardial infarction has as its objectives a reduction both in death rates from subsequent myocardial infarction and in the extent of invalidism following a clinical episode of this illness. The purpose of this chapter is to present information both on the nature of the various outcomes that might be observed in patients after myocardial infarction and on the extent to which these outcomes have been observed in a selection of clinical studies.

To speak of outcome after myocardial infarction as a simple, unitary phenomenon is to badly oversimplify a distinctly multifaceted process. It might be said that each individual has his or her own unique outcome after an episode of myocardial infarction and that no two patterns of outcome in different individuals are precisely the same. This claim to wide individual differences is well documented in the literature (Byrne, Whyte, & Butler, 1981) and underscores the fact that outcomes after myocardial infarction are determined by factors more wide ranging than the simple extent of coronary-artery blockage or myocardial tissue loss.

The variable that most commonly interacts with the multitude of factors bearing on outcome after myocardial infarction is time. In the immediate sense, the time elapsing between the recognition of symptoms and the initiation of help-seeking behavior has been shown to relate to short-term mortality rates (Surwit et al., 1982), though more broadly speaking the whole range of outcomes that might eventuate after acute myocardial infarction can be related to the time since the original event. In fact, it has been noted (Finlayson & McEwen, 1977) that the entire range of possible outcomes can not be considered to have run its full course until about four years after the initial hospitalization.

For reasons largely to do with the vulnerability of the myocardium and the coronary circulation, outcomes which emerge in the first hours and days after myocardial infarction are almost exclusively within the cardiovascular realm and typically take the form of coronary mortality. Emotional responses to illness are usually transient at this point and must await consolidation before they can be considered as a component of outcome. Similarly, the real pattern of occupational and social outcomes can not become apparent until the patient has been discharged from hospital and has re-entered the working and social environments. The simplest categorization of this temporal sequence would involve (a) the acute phase in the first days following onset of symptoms, where the cardiovascular system is vulnerable to physiological complications, (b) the recovery phase, usually encompassing the whole period of hospitalization, where cardiological complications remain a cause for concern but where emotional responses to illness begin to consolidate, (c) the short-term rehabilitation phase sometimes bounded by return to work, where the process of readjustment to social, family, and occupational roles begins and where nonmedical intervention is most frequently seen, and (d) the long-term rehabilitation phase extending, perhaps, over some years after hospitalization, where the process of adjustment is tested in the real world. Within this context, the patient who survives a myocardial infarction sufficiently long to be admitted to a coronary-care unit is faced with a potential set of both immediate and short-term outcomes of a strictly medical nature. These range from an uncomplicated recovery and an uneventful return to normal life through to physiological disruptions to the heart and circulatory system that might ultimately lead to death. Should the patient be fortunate enough to avoid the more life threatening or disabling medical consequences of myocardial infarction, he or she is still faced in the longer term with a variety of occupational, social, and emotional outcomes, some of which are far from satisfactory. Some patients are able to return to work relatively rapidly and, what is more, are able to fulfill the same occupational demands existing before the myocardial infarction. Others either have great difficulty in returning to work at all or, if they are able to rejoin the work force, are nonetheless compelled to change the nature and demands of their jobs so as to compensate for the decreased cardiac capacity occasioned by the myocardial infarction. Even if the patient makes an uneventful medical recovery and is able to resume active employment, he or she may be burdened by protracted emotional distress, typically anxiety and depression which, though perhaps evident soon after illness onset, may consolidate with time. Moreover, uncertainty and concern regarding physical capacity and the probability of a further episode of illness may substantially hinder the patient's complete return to an adequate social, family, and sexual life.

There are two messages to be distilled from this preamble. Firstly, outcome following myocardial infarction must be regarded as a manifestly complex phenomenon. Indeed, at least three aspects of outcome must be considered to contribute to this overall pattern. Survivors of one myocardial infarction may, in the course of time, sustain a further myocardial infarction that they may or may not survive. They might also experience a variety of potentially dangerous and unpleasant medical complications which, while they do not amount to recurrent myocardial infarction, can still result in discomfort, disability, and protracted incapacity. Thus, outcome must be defined, in part, by cardiological status after myocardial infarction. Cay, Vetter, Philip, and Dugard (1973) were, however, led to comment that for the majority of survivors of myocardial infarction, a successful outcome was defined by "return to work without loss of status and earnings." Thus, the resumption of a productive life style-must also be regarded as a defining component of outcome. Moreover, as Mayou, Foster, and Williamson (1978) have pointed out, even when medical and occupational outcomes are judged on objective grounds to be satisfactory, the patient may still experience quite substantial levels of emotional and social incapacity.

The essentially multidimensional nature of outcome after myocardial infarction is now well recognized. Major studies that were concerned a decade ago only with recurrent infarction or return to work are now concerned also with whether the patient is burdened with undue emotional distress, or has been able to resume a fulfilling social life (Croog & Levine, 1977; Finlayson & McEwen, 1977). The recognition of "quality of life" issues as legitimate indices of outcome after myocardial infarction has expanded the realms of patient management to a very substantial extent.

The second point to be taken from the preceding discussion has to do with the time course of outcome after myocardial infarction. Most studies of outcome have reported on patients' recovery and rehabilitation between three and 12 months after the illness. Finlayson and McEwen (1977) have, however, pointed out that outcome after myocardial infarction is a developing and protracted process that is often not completely resolved until some years after the original illness. In this respect it is important to note (Byrne, 1982) that some aspects of outcome that are of particular importance at one stage during the process of recovery and rehabilitation are perhaps of lesser importance or overshadowed by other aspects of outcome later in the process. Thus, in the early stages of recovery the overriding concern is for the physical well-being of the patient, while in the later stages of rehabilitation, the medical status of the patient usually having been resolved by that point, the patient's social and occupational adjustment become the more relevant foci for attention.

It is important to note that while myocardial infarction is a life-threatening illness with the distinct risk of death and disability, the prognosis for those who survive the physiological insult of the clinical event can be very good indeed. Moreover, with appropriate intervention, both medical and behavioral, this prognosis has the potential for noticeable improvement. However, in a major review of psychosocial aspects of recovery from coronary heart disease, Doehrman (1977) concluded:

> There is little question that coronary heart disease results in the temporary disruption of normal psychological and social functioning. Long lasting emotional distress, familial problems and occupational maladjustment are observed in a significant minority of patients. (p. 199)

2. PATTERNS OF CARDIOLOGICAL OUTCOME

The majority of epidemiological studies of outcome after myocardial infarction have used mortality or morbidity arising from subsequent myocardial infarction as the major end point. This choice is easily understandable in that such events constitute convenient, concrete, and well-recognized end points in a clinical process and are subject to ready confirmation by medical records and death-certificate data. It is also understandable in the context that medical attention is most frequently directed at maximizing survival and minimizing cardiological complications after myocardial infarction and, as Pole et al. (1977) have pointed out, precise information on the natural history of survival after myocardial infarction is essential for the success of this medical task.

There is considerable between-study variation both in reported mortality and morbidity from subsequent myocardial infarction after an initial episode of this illness (Shapiro, Weinblatt, Frank, & Sager, 1969) though some of this is to be understood in terms of differing methods of case ascertainment or criteria for the diagnosis of myocardial infarction and variability in the length of the follow-up period reported on. The nature of the populations under investigation is also an important variable in assessing patterns of cardiological outcome after myocardial infarction since subsequent morbidity and mortality may be related to the delay between recognition of symptoms and admission to hospital, the patient's age (Pole et al., 1977), severity of the myocardial infarction (Norris, Caughey, Deeming, Mercer, & Scott, 1970) and the continuing level of standard-risk factors. Studies on cardiological outcome must, therefore, be viewed within these interpretive constraints.

Data from an extensive list of studies could be cited to demonstrate the overall pattern of cardiological outcomes after myocardial infarction. Those presented in this chapter were chosen on the grounds that they provided a broad overview of the basic variables (age, follow-up period, and so on) bearing on outcome rates. Additionally, most studies chosen had psychological contributions to outcome as at least one of the main emphases of investigation. The studies are, however, representative of the field of outcome research after myocardial infarction, and there is no reason to believe that other epidemiological data on this clinical process would present a different picture.

In a study involving admissions to the coronary-care unit of a general hospital in Scotland, mortality from all causes in the first 12 months following myocardial infarction was reported to be 18% (Cay et al., 1973). The overwhelming reason for subsequent mortality was, however, a further episode of myocardial infarction. It is worth noting, however, that this sample of patients had an average age somewhat higher than is generally seen in studies of outcome. In another Scottish study, this time centered on the Dundee area, Finlayson and McEwen (1977) noted a 12-month mortality from all causes after first myocardial infarction of 14.5%, once more taken up primarily by further heart disease. The sample in this instance was slightly younger, on average, than that just cited.

Croog and Levine (1977), studying a North American population, reported a 12-month morbidity from survived myocardial infarction of 14.9% in a large sample of males initially admitted to hospital with a first, well-documented myocardial infarction. In addition, a 12-month mortality, also from subsequent myocardial infarction, was found for a further 4.5% of the sample. Patients in this study were all males under 60 years on admission to the study who had experienced an uncomplicated period of recovery during hospitalization. As such, they would be expected to enjoy relatively good prospects for long-term survival.

An investigation of a similar population from the Midwestern United States (Marmor, Geltman, Schechtman, Sobel, & Roberts, 1982) revealed a nine-month rate of recurrent myocardial infarction, survived or otherwise, among a large sample of survivors of a first episode of that illness, as ranging between 8% and 43%. The important variable in explaining this difference was that of the site of myocardial infarction, with subendocardial infarctions endowing a greater risk of recurrence than transmural ones.

In Finland, where overall rates of first myocardial infarction are high relative to world standards, cumulative coronary mortality over three years among a large sample of survivors of an initial episode of myocardial infarction was shown to be 29.4%, of which 14.4% was taken up in the form of sudden death, mostly occurring in the first six months after the initial event (Kallio, Hamalainen, Hakkila, & Luurila, 1979). All patients were aged less than 65 years on admission to the study and their hospitalization marked their first heart attack.

By contrast, in Japan, where overall rates of myocardial infarction are relatively low, Takeuchi (1983) followed a large cohort of survivors of first myocardial infarction over a period of five years and seven months and found the cumulative mortality rate from subsequent cardiac disease to be 14.7%.

Australian data fall reasonably close to those from North America, as one might expect from cultures sharing a wide range of attitudes and attributes. Byrne, Whyte & Butler (1981) examined a cohort of survivors of a first, well-documented myocardial infarction eight months after the initial event and found a morbidity rate from subsequent myocardial infarction of 19.6%. A further 6.0% of the sample suffered a heart attack in this time period and did not survive. These data are closely similar to those reported by Croog and Levine (1977) resulting, perhaps, from a strong resemblance in the attributes defining the two samples. A re-examination of these Australian patients 24 months after the initial myocardial infarction revealed that a further 25% had suffered a subsequent heart attack, whether survived or not, in the period between follow-up (Byrne, 1982).

In a separate Australian community, a longitudinal study of survivors of uncomplicated, first myocardial infarction reported rates of sudden cardiac death six months, one year, and three years after the initial event as 2.7%, 4.5%, and 7.3% respectively. Patients who had experienced a subsequent but survived episode of myocardial infarction in these follow-up periods accounted for a further 3.4%, 8.2% and 18.5% of the cohort (Jelinek, McDonald, Ryan, Ziffer, Clemens, & Gerloff, 1982). While these rates, particularly in the earlier period following myocardial infarction, are somewhat lower than those reported by Byrne et al. (1981) it should be noted that this study did not select for patients with uncomplicated initial infarctions, and patients may therefore have been at a marginally greater risk of subsequent heart attack.

Data from these studies are summarized in Table 2.1 here where it can be seen that rates of subsequent coronary morbidity and mortality show a pattern of considerable diversity for which one can look to a range of explanations. Firstly, the length of the follow-up period will bear strongly on the outcome rates reported by the various studies. Clearly, a study that follows patients over a long period of time will accumulate greater rates of recurrent myocardial infarction than one that terminates data collection only months after the initial event, though it is equally clear (Kallio et al., 1979) that the greatest rates of subsequent morbidity and mortality are to be seen nearer rather than further away from the first heart attack. Secondly, the mean age of the sample is crucial in the interpretation of data on cardiological outcome. According to Willerson et al. (1982):

Table 2.1. Data from Selected Studies Illustrating Morbidity and Mortality Rates Following Survived Myocardial Infarction

Source	Follow-up Interval	Morbidity Rate	Mortality Rate
Cay et al. (1973)	12 months	NA	18.0%[*]
Pole et al. (1976)	12 months	NA	14.5%[*]
	5 years	NA	33.0%[*]
	9 years	NA	48.0%[*] (cumulative)
Finlayson and McEwen (1977)	12 month	NA	14.5%[*]
Croog and Levine (1977)	12 months	14.9%[+]	4.5%[+]
Kallio et al. (1979)	3 years	NA	29.4%[+]
Byrne et al. (1980)	8 months	19.6%[+]	6.9%[+]
Byrne (1982)	2 years	25%[+] (combined rate)	
Jelinek et al. (1982)	6 months	3.4%[+]	2.7%[+]
	12 months	8.2%[+]	4.5%[+]
	3 years	18.5%[+]	7.3%[+]
Takeuchi (1983)	5 years	NA	14.7%[+]

[*]Mortality from all causes
[+] Mortality or morbidity from subsequent myocardial infarction only

In general, if the patient is less than 50 years of age at the time of the initial infarction, the annual mortality rate is approximately 5%. If the patient is over 50 years of age, the mortality rate is approximately double. If a patient survives one year following infarction, there is a 75% chance he will survive 5. If he survives for five years following infarction there is approximately a 50% chance he will live 15 years. (p. 292)

Most studies have restricted the age of patients in samples to 65 years or less. Some, however, have allowed the mean age of samples to rise by including consecutive admissions to coronary-care units regardless of age. Since the incidence of myocardial infarction is age related in any event, and since degenerative disease of the heart and circulation increases with age, it is not surprising to find, as a general effect, that samples where the age range is restricted to those under 65 years at onset of the original myocardial infarction tend to show lower subsequent morbidity and mortality rates than do samples that include older subjects. (The same effect can be observed, incidentally, for return to work; because if a patient has retired at 65, resumption of occupation is no longer a pertinent index of outcome.)

The certainty of diagnosis necessary for inclusion into the study must, thirdly, be taken into account in interpreting outcome data. Stringent diagnostic criteria, leading to homogeneous samples of patients with myocardial infarction, tend to result in higher subsequent morbidity and mortality rates than when a loose set of criteria are applied to patients on admission to longitudinal studies. In fact, the World Health Organization has specified diagnostic criteria providing diagnoses of both unequivocal and equivocal myocardial infarction for use in collaborative studies initiated by this body (World Health Organization, 1973). Similarly, and lastly, the certainty of diagnosis on follow-up must enter into the interpretation of outcome rates. Some studies express mortality in terms of deaths from all causes, others from equivocal myocardial infarction, and others still record only definite heart attack. This produces a clear gradient of outcome rates over the several possibilities of outcome, so these categories should never be treated as equivalent. This latter point is possibly more critical when morbidity (a survived illness event) is used as the index of outcome, because the latitude for diagnostic errors is greater. Regrettably, few studies quote, or even know, attrition rates from the cohort; this has the distinct potential to obscure results, as the group which becomes unavailable for follow-up is likely to have a high representation from those who have suffered a further illness event, either survived or not.

These issues bearing on the interpretation of outcome data should not be confused with factors determining patterns of cardiological outcome following myocardial infarction. They are considered in Chapter 4. The former do underscore, however, the need for population—as opposed to clinical stuty—data, so as to provide the most accurate estimates of these indices of outcome. In this respect, the coronary-care register study of Pole et al. (1977) provides a useful illustration.

The methodology of this study has been touched on in the previous chapter in relation to incidence rates for myocardial infarction. More pertinent to the present discussion, the data also provide a careful and complete account of the clinical course after myocardial infarction within a total population. The one-year incidence of acute myocardial infarction within a study population of 630,000 was 740/100,000 in men aged 30 to 69, and 220/100,000 in women of the same age range. These data provide as complete as possible a reflection of the experience of myocardial infarction within the specified community and are therefore to be seen as accurate baseline data.

Further investigation revealed that 26% of men and 21% of women died before reaching hospital, while an additional 16% of men and 17% of women died during the period of hospitalization. By contrast, only 5% of men and of women died in the period between discharge from hospital and the end of the 12-month follow-up. Deaths from subsequent myocardial infarction were, as expected, strongly related to the patient's age, with younger patients showing substantially lower death rates than older ones. It can be seen that the bulk of the overall 47% one-year mortality in men and the 43% mortality in women occurred in the first days after the onset of the initial illness. A finer breakdown of these data (Martin, Thompson, Armstrong, Hobbs, & DeClerk, 1983) indicated combined death rates in the first 24 hours to be 23%, with an additional death rate in the first 28 days after myocardial infarction of 15%. The crucial importance of the first hours and days for long-term survival after myocardial infarction can not, therefore, be underestimated.

Other data have suggested a somewhat higher death rate, particularly in the first hour after the onset of symptoms, with around 50% of patients not surviving to be admitted to hospital (Surwit et al., 1982), though there is evidence that this figure has been dramatically reduced with the availability of coronary-care ambulance facilities (Willerson et al, 1982). While mortality at this stage can not, of course, be considered an aspect of cardiological outcome (it is part of the clinical course of the initial myocardial infarction), the behavioral factors bearing on it are relevant to events in the longer term. One of the primary reasons underlying death at this stage is the failure to treat potentially reversible ventricular fibrillation, and of the several explanations for this, misidentification of symptoms and denial of their significance by the patient are prominent. That is, patients tend to ignore or misattribute even quite severe symptoms at the onset of myocardial infarction, so that medical treatment is delayed past the time when it can reasonably be of use. In a review of studies on delay in the recognition of cardiac symptoms, Surwit et al. (1982) said:

> Psychologically, sudden cardiac deaths appear to be the consequence of faulty decision making on the part of the patient, physician and family, which is in turn related to a pathological use of denial by persons wishing to avoid the compelling realities of traumatic illness.

It is very likely that, having once used this potentially fatal means of psychological defense, individuals will return to it in the face of future episodes of the same distressing and frightening cardiac symptoms.

3. PATTERNS OF OCCUPATIONAL OUTCOME

Occupational outcome after myocardial infarction figures almost as prominently in the clinical and epidemiological literature as cardiological outcome. This is an important index because, while the medical prognosis for most patients who survive the initial days of myocardial infarction is quite good, these same patients may for many reasons experience considerable difficulties and delays in returning to work. Thus for many patients the real evidence of a totally successful recovery from myocardial infarction is apparent in a "return to work without loss of status and earning" (Cay et al., 1973).

Aspects of occupational outcome, like those of cardiological outcome, are attractive in both clinical and epidemiological studies because they form well-defined and quantifiable points of progress and achievement through the processes of recovery and rehabilitation. In general terms, occupational outcome can be divided into three distinct areas. The first of these is return to work, and can be defined simply by whether or not the patient is able to return to active and productive employment in return for wages or salary. The second aspect has to do with delay in returning to work and is measured as the time elapsing between the onset of myocardial infarction and the resumption of such active employment. The third aspect concerns whether return to work signals a return to the same level of job status and activity as existed prior to myocardial infarction or whether the occurrence of the illness and its medical or social consequences demand that the patient accept a job involving decreased activity or diminished status and responsibility.

The interrelationships between these aspects of occupational outcome are complex. It is possible, for example, for a patient on surviving a myocardial infarction to rapidly resume employment at premorbid levels of activity and then to find the demands of the job sufficiently taxing for retirement or a change to a lower level of employment to become necessary. Moreover, such decisions are not always left with the patients themselves, but are often strongly influenced by relatives and employees. Outcome data indicating an initially rapid return to work may, therefore, be confounded by subsequent difficulties, either physical or personal, resulting in eventual termination or modification of employment. The sociological aspects of this process have been comprehensively addressed by Finlayson and McEwen (1977). It is important to note then, that influences more extensive than the cardiological status of the patient and the opinions of the patient's physicians bear on occupational outcome after myocardial infarction.

The data on rates of return to work after myocardial infarction and the ability to maintain a level of activity and job status identical to that which existed prior to illness, vary considerably from study to study. In an early investigation, Master and Dack (1940) reported that only 59% of patients who had experienced a first myocardial infarction were able to return to work at any time after the illness. This may, among other things, reflect the somewhat conservative attitudes held by physicians four decades ago on the ability of survivors of myocardial infarction to resume an active employment status, because the social conditions prevailing at the time would have endowed the physicians' opinions with considerable authority. Sixteen years later, Crain and Missall (1956), reporting on the retrospective examination of medical records relative to 184 male survivors of myocardial infarction, found that 82% of patients were eventually able to resume active employment. This represents an advance on the earlier data, and perhaps reflects a progression of medical attitudes, though it is not possible to discount differences in the two samples as being responsible for the variation in rates. This point is perhaps illuminated by the finding of Morris (1959) that eventual rates of return to work were influenced by the severity of the myocardial infarction, with 65% of survivors of mild infarction eventually resuming their jobs but only 33% of survivors of severe infarction able to do so. In a large study of the psychological and occupational consequence of myocardial infarction, Cay et al. (1973) reported a four-month return-to-work rate of 36%, with a 12-month rate climbing to 77%. The four-month return-to-work rate contrasts somewhat with a three-month rate of 76% reported for a sample of Irish subjects by Mulcahy (1976), though this may reflect differences in the age structure as well as other aspects of the two samples. Finlayson and McEwen (1977) reported a six-month return-to-work rate of 77% in a sample of British male subjects, while Croog and Levine (1977) in a 12-month follow-up of male survivors of myocardial infarction in the U.S.A., found a one-year return-to-work rate of 76%.

In another follow-up of male survivors of myocardial infarction, Byrne et al. (1980) found that 85% of their patients had returned to work at eight-month follow-up, though this had declined to 66% when these patients were followed up 24 months after discharge from hospital (Byrne, 1982). These data illustrate the point that occupational outcome after myocardial infarction may not be totally resolved over a relatively short follow-up period, and a longer period of follow-up may reveal less satisfactory patterns of ultimate outcome than those evident in the first year after myocardial infarction (Finlayson & McEwen, 1977). The initially superior rates of return to work reported by Byrne et al. (1980) relative to data emerging from other studies may simply reflect the fact that this sample was restricted to men under 65 years of age at the onset of illness (mean age was 54 years) who were all in active employment and who had experienced their first myocardial infarction. A summary of these data can be seen in Table 2.2.

A more complete view of return to work following myocardial infarction can be gained from an inspection of the temporal patterns which this takes on. Byrne

Table 2.2. Data from Selected Studies Illustrating Rates of Return to Work
Following Survived Myocardial Infarction

Source	Follow-up Interval	Return Rate
Crain and Missal (1956)	NA	82%
Morris (1959)	NA	65% (Mild MI)
		33% (Severe MI)
Pell and D'Alonzo (1963)	12 months	80% (White-collar jobs)
		70% (Blue-collar jobs)
Weinblatt et al. (1966)	18 months	95% (White-collar jobs)
		85% (Blue-collar jobs)
Johnson (1966)	12 months	85%
Cay et al. (1973)	4 months	36%
	12 months	77%
Mulcahy (1976)	3 months	76%
Croog and Levine (1977)	12 months	76%
Finlayson and McEwen (1977)	6 months	77%
Byrne et al. (1980)	8 months	85%

et al. (1980) found that 14% of their sample had in fact returned to work within one month of myocardial infarction. A further 74% returned to work between one and three months after illness while only 12% of patients who would eventually return to work in eight months took more than four months to do so. These data are presented in Fig. 2.1. Evidence such as this would indicate that while rates of return to work are often presented over a relatively long follow-up period, the process of return to work need not be protracted, and most patients who will ultimately do so seem able to resume active employment within three months of illness onset. The data are not, however, in complete agreement in this respect, and a contrasting view from the work of Cay et al. (1973) can also be seen in Fig. 2.1.

This evidence notwithstanding, it is important to remember that rates of return to work apparent in the relatively short term after myocardial infarction may not prevail in the longer term, with patients who initially resumed active employment, perhaps prematurely and against medical advice, being then compelled, for medical or psychosocial reasons, to change the nature of their work, return to periods of medical leave, or seek early retirement. In this respect, there is some evidence that the nature of the occupation exerts an influence on the patient's success in resuming active employment. Pell and D'Alonzo (1963) found the 12 month return-to-work rate among white-collar patients to be 80% while only 70% of their blue-collar colleagues were able to resume employment in the same time period. Similarly, Weinblatt, Shapiro, Frank, & Sager (1966) found that 95% of white-collar survivors of myocardial infarction were able to return to work after 18 months, while only 85% of blue-collar patients were able

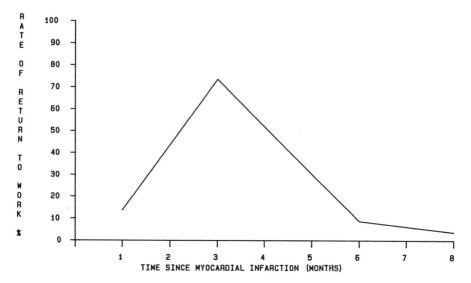

Figure 2.1 Time taken to return to work among survivors of myocardial infarction actively employed at the onset of illness (from Byrne, Whyte, & Butler, Journal of Psychosomatic Research, Vol. 25, 1981).

to do so. It might be argued from this that the physical demands of blue collar as opposed to white collar occupations, whether actual or perceived, sufficiently challenge a vulnerable and incapacitated myocardium that blue-collar workers are less able to resume employment than are white-collar employees. The situation is likely to be more complex than this however. Byrne et al. (1980) categorized the nature of occupations into the three classes of "sedentary," "light physical," and "moderate/heavy physical" and found no statisical association between the physical demands of the occupation and rates of return to work.

It is clear, then, that a variety of influences bear on a person's ability to resume active and unimpeded employment following myocardial infarction. Age is certainly a factor, with older patients being less likely to return to work than younger ones. This may be due to a tendency among older patients to focus upon the illness as a convenient and acceptable reason for retirement. It may also be due, however, to the possibility that older patients are subject to more medical complications following myocardial infarction, including recurrent illness, than are younger patients, necessitating the adoption of a less demanding life-style. There is some evidence that the nature of the occupation exerts an influence on return to work, though in view of the results of Byrne et al. (1981), it is unlikely that this is entirely a function of the physical demands of the job. It may be bound up in a more complex way with the observation that patients in blue-collar occupations tend to exhibit significantly more anxiety in response to myocardial

30

infarction than do patients in white-collar occupations (Byrne, 1980). While there is little to link this reported anxiety with specific concerns, irrational fears regarding the effects of physical effort on the heart may be as apparent as more realistic views of residual cardiac capacity among patients recovering from myocardial infarction.

In this respect, however, it is not always the patients themselves or their medical advisers who hold the power of decision in returning to work. It is becoming more common for employers or employment policies to play a role in this process. In societies where work performance and job pressure are accorded a degree of occupational prominence, and where litigation for work-related illness is becoming more common, employers are frequently reluctant to encourage employees who have suffered a myocardial infarction to return to work, even when the recovery has been cardiologically uneventful. This may reflect the often mistaken belief that myocardial infarction portends a prolonged physical incapacity and a low probability of resuming previous work performance (Mulcahy, 1976; Doehrman, 1977).

The severity of the myocardial infarction as measured by a variety of medical parameters bears a clear relation to medical prognosis (Norris, Caughey, Deeming, Mercer, & Scott, 1970); though, except where the illness is very serious, the recent evidence is equivocal respecting its influence on occupational outcome. Mulcahy (1976) in fact recommends a return to previous levels of occupation regardless of the objective severity of the myocardial infarction.

4. PATTERNS OF PSYCHOSOCIAL OUTCOME

While medical recovery and the resumption of active employment are clearly the most prominent measures in studies of outcome after myocardial infarction, the discussion would be incomplete without mention of one further manifestation of this process—namely psychosocial adjustment. Measures of this aspect of outcome are conspicuously absent in most studies, and several reasons might be advanced to explain this. Aspects of psychosocial outcome are frequently more difficult both to define and to measure than are aspects of either cardiological or occupational outcome, and their absence from major epidemiological studies of outcome may reflect this perceived problem. Indeed, mention of psychosocial outcome implies a concern with so-called quality-of-life issues, and such sociological matters are frequently not thought to be the proper substance of medical research. Psychosocial outcome certainly encompasses a large and diverse set of end points or steps in the patient's progress, ranging from poorly defined measures of self-perceived well-being through expressions of personal satisfaction with progress to more concrete, psychometrically assessed indices of personal adjustment and social integration. As such, the problems posed by the selection of appropriate and clinically useful measures, together with the obvious difficulties of accuracy and contamination of self-reported data in these areas, represent substantial methodological dilemmas in research strategies. However, the few studies to have investigated this area have revealed a set of potential difficulties for the survivor of myocardial infarction that are too extensive to ignore.

Doehrman (1977) commented with some certainty that an episode of myocardial infarction produces for most patients a temporary disruption of normal psychological and social functioning. For a significant minority it results in protracted emotional distress, familial problems, and social maladjustment. In a similar light, Mayou et al. (1978) were led to conclude that social disability following myocardial infarction was of far greater proportions than had previously been described in the literature and was, furthermore, largely unrelated to the severity of the myocardial infarction. It is important, therefore, that any chapter on outcome after myocardial infarction should include a discussion of the psychosocial consequences of this illness.

Finlayson and McEwen (1977), in a study of 76 married men who had survived a first myocardial infarction, reported considerable social disruption in their patients' lives up to four years after the initial myocardial infarction. Almost half their sample (49%) had experienced a decrease in social activities four years after myocardial infarction relative to the level of social activity prior to illness. Moreover, 12% of their sample claimed that they had not been able to achieve a stable pattern of social life involving the maintenance of social networks even four years after myocardial infarction.

Mayou and his colleagues (Mayou, 1979; Mayou et al. 1978a and 1978b) conducted three successive interviews on each of 100 patients who had survived a first myocardial infarction. These were soon after their admission to hospital and then at two months and one year after hospital discharge. The focus of this study had to do with the nature and time course of psychosocial adjustment after myocardial infarction. Psychological distress was still prominent one year after myocardial infarction, with 64% of patients reporting moderate to marked states of anxiety, depression, and associated affective symptoms. Myocardial infarction seemed also to make considerable inroads into leisure activity, with 30% of patients feeling compelled to make major changes in their levels of leisure activity and a further 36% making smaller changes following illness. By contrast with the report of Finlayson and McEwen (1977), patterns of social interaction were not markedly affected by myocardial infarction, though 35% of patients reported a decrease in the level of social activities while 12% felt that their social life was less satisfactory following illness than before. Such patterns of social disruption which became apparent at two months after myocardial infarction seemed to persist into the longer term, so that it may be possible to predict chronic and protracted difficulties on the basis of relatively immediate responses to illness (Mayou, 1984). On these grounds, Mayou was able to recommend that systematic clinical assessment during admission or shortly after discharge from hospital might detect patients most in danger of protracted social disability and point to those most in need of specific psychological intervention.

In overviewing these data Mayou (1979) was careful to point out that previous views of psychosocial disability following myocardial infarction had been too simplistic and it was evident from the present data that each aspect of psychosocial state must be considered separately. Moreover, it seemed that the wide variation in patterns of psychosocial disability following myocardial infarction could be accounted for, in part, by the influence of observed or inferred patterns of premorbid adjustment evident for any patient and by the simultaneous occurrence of life events during the periods of recovery and rehabilitation. The role of the premorbid psychological state and of the continuous intrusion of life events after the illness as contributors to both cardiological and psychosocial outcome have more recently been highlighted in other work (Byrne, 1979; Byrne et al. 1981).

One crucial point emerging from this work (Mayou et al., 1978b) had to do with the effect of myocardial infarction on patients' spouses. These authors found that affective distress evident among patients was reciprocally evident in their spouses, and patterns of social disability to be seen among patients were reflected in the levels of spouses' social activity. This influence has previously been observed by Finlayson and McEwen (1977) and points to the need for spouse involvement in the clinical management of survivors of myocardial infarction.

Byrne (1982), too, reported on the patterns of psychosocial outcome in survivors of myocardial infarction. In line with the findings of Mayou this study revealed substantial levels of self-reported psychosocial difficulties following myocardial infarction. Between 20% and 30% of all patients reported some form of emotional distress, most prominently depression, in the eight months after myocardial infarction. More than half of the sample complained of an overwhelming sense of limitation in their physical activity after illness, while 20% of the sample expressed a perceived need for rest greatly in excess of that felt prior to illness. Social disruption too, was evident, with 23% of patients complaining of a change in social life for the worse after myocardial infarction and 25% of patients reporting a substantially diminished level of social activity. This reported disruption of social activities was similar in character to a response observed soon after the onset of myocardial infarction, where the same group of patients had reported disturbances in social relationships secondary to feelings of affective distress. In view of the known associations between mood state and social integration (Henderson, Byrne, & Duncan Jones, 1981), it is possible that a failure of social reintegration after myocardial infarction is as much related to prevailing anxiety and depression as it is to any physical incapacity occasioned by the illness. Interestingly, though at odds with the findings of Mayou, only 5% of the sample reported difficulties in spouse adjustment and reciprocal anxiety within the family.

Essentially similar patterns of social dislocation after myocardial infarction can be seen in the data of Wiklund, Sanne, Vedin, and Wilhelmsson (1984) on middle-aged Swedish males. Emotional distress, self-reported symptoms of cardiovascular disease, disruption of social relationships and leisure activities, emergence of overprotective attitudes by the spouse, and diminished sexual activity were all evident in survivors of myocardial infarction to degrees in excess of those characterizing premorbid functioning. These features were apparent two months after the onset of illness and persisted, largely unchanged, up to a year following hospital discharge. Failure to achieve social and psychological adjustment both at two months and one year after myocardial infarction was unrelated to the objective severity of the heart attack, indicating that individual perceptions of cardiovascular damage rather than actual levels of cardiac incapacity are the more important determinants of social disruption in the long term.

Therefore, while data on psychosocial outcome after myocardial infarction do involve indices or outcome which, to traditional epidemiological investigation, are somewhat "soft," the prevalence of such measures of outcome is quite widespread and would seem to form a legitimate area of interest for those concerned with the consequences of myocardial infarction. Since these measures of outcome are also essentially social and behavioral in nature, they are particularly important to a consideration of the behavioral management of the cardiac patient and should not be neglected. The issue of measurement of patterns of psychosocial outcome will, of course, be more controversial than measurement of cardiological or occupational outcome, as the former requires both subjective self-report by the patient and a degree of judgment on the part of the clinical interviewer. Such data as these should, however, be familiar to those involved with the care of patients experiencing behavioral and emotional problems.

5.   OVERVIEW

It is clear that the once prevailing view of myocardial infarction as an event signaling imminent death or irrecoverable disability is no longer tenable. The evidence would suggest that of those who survive the life-threatening arrhythmias of the first hours after myocardial infarction, between 70% and 80% (taken across all studies) will continue to survive for 12 months. The first days after the onset of illness involve a moderately high risk that the patient will succumb either to a second heart attack or to heart failure or disturbances of heart rhythm to which the heart is vulnerable following myocardial infarction. While further coronary events resulting in death or progressive loss of cardiac capacity will occur after the acute phase, the chance of these events decreases with time elapsing since the initial attack. This is particularly evident in younger patients.

The termination of this acute phase, in which physiological events dominate the clinical picture, allows the emergence of other aspects of outcome as it signals the beginning of the period in which patients will attempt the process of return to work and social reintegration. This period is more protracted; and while it is rapidly and easily accomplished by some, it is a time during which others experience great difficulties. Both return to work and social adjustment may be complicated by the occurrence of a further myocardial infarction or continued cardiac disability in a small group of patients, particularly the older ones. For the younger ones, however, it would seem that success in resuming work and in social adjustment are shaped as much by personal perceptions of the severity of the heart attack and its medical consequences as by objective levels of cardiac incapacity. Thus, in the absence of appropriate intervention, the processes of occupational and social rehabilitation may take place over years and not months. In this respect, it is apparent that the physical survival from myocardial infarction represents only the beginning, after which the individual patient remains subject to continued problems involving resumption of work and the re-establishment of social roles and responsibilities. These latter indices of outcome appear, however-er, at least partly under the control of premorbid patterns of personality, thought and behavior; and, as such, are potentially modifiable by means of psychological strategies of management.

CHAPTER 3

Psychological Responses To Myocardial Infarction

1. THE EXPERIENCE OF ILLNESS

Life crises inevitably produce emotional consequences. The experience of myocardial infarction is a major crisis for most individuals and in the short term the most typically observed response to this event will be emotional distress in one of its various forms. Myocardial infarction will assume different cognitive meanings for different people (Byrne & Whyte, 1978); however, the observable characteristics of the illness experience are essentially invariant. Firstly, it is a life-threatening experience which, in some individuals, will inititate thoughts, attitudes, and even preoccupations about the nearness of death (Cay et al., 1972). Secondly, the onset of symptoms will herald the beginning of a potentially long period of recovery and rehabilitation and will imply, for some, the possibility of protracted disability (Finlayson & McEwen, 1977). Thirdly, the acute phase of myocardial infarction may bring with it a period of pain and physical discomfort and an unavoidable dependence on the attentions of others (Byrne & Whyte, 1979). Finally, enforced occupation of an intensive coronary-care unit with its necessary but mysterious technology, and with the potential to witness medical emergencies in other victims of the same illness will for a significant minority of people constitute what has been called a psychological hazard (Hackett, Cassem, & Wishnie, 1968). The collective actions of these factors, while they might be mediated by a range of influences including individual patterns of personality, past experience with myocardial infarction either personal or vicarious, the degree of information communicated by physician to patient about the nature of the illness, the sociocultural expectations regarding myocardial infarction inherent in a given society and levels of simultaneous life stress and social support, will act to produce a range of affective, behavioral, and cognitive responses to myocardial infarction which will bear on immediate progress during the stages of medical recovery and will most likely influence the long-term outcome for any individual patient. These responses can be discussed at two levels. On the one hand, they reflect emotional distress, perhaps intense but essentially time limited, representing a realistic recognition of the presence of serious illness. On the other hand, emotional distress may achieve an intensity and duration out of proportion to the threat occasioned by the myocardial infarction, and patterns of thought and behaviour at odds with adaptation to the demands of the illness event.

2. AFFECTIVE DISTURBANCE AFTER MYOCARDIAL INFARCTION

The experience of emotional symptoms of substantial proportions is not an uncommon, immediate response to myocardial infarction (Cay et al., 1973) and in a certain percentage of patients, differing from one study to another but always sufficiently large to be of clinical importance, these affective symptoms can be both prolonged and disabling (Doehrman, 1977). Estimates of the prevalence of severe emotional reactions to myocardial infarction vary, though a recent study employing a structured psychiatric interview to assess clinically significant disturbance indicated that 35% of a consecutive series of 100 male survivors of myocardial infarction exhibited conspicuous psychiatric morbidity within the first week after admission to hospital (Lloyd & Cawley, 1982). Of these, 16 patients were found to have been psychiatrically disturbed before the heart attack and their symptoms persisted throughout a 12 month follow-up period. By contrast, the patients whose emotional symptoms appeared to have been precipitated by the myocardial infarction tended to have transient difficulties, and few if any protracted problems.

A series of reports by Cay and her colleagues in Edinburgh examined in more detail the nature and course of symptoms of psychological disturbance evident in survivors of myocardial infarction. Overall prevalence rate for emotional disturbance was similar to that reported by Lloyd and Cawley (1982), though disturbance was detected in this case by means of a symptom questionnaire (the Personal Disturbance Scale of the Symptom Sign Inventory). Using this technique it was found that 43% of patients who had suffered a first myocardial infarction and 27% of patients who had suffered a subsequent myocardial infarction reported borderline symptoms of overt psychological disorder. More severe symptoms attracting the label "psychiatric disturbance" were evident in a further 30% of patients with first myocardial infarction, and this rose to 42% of patients with subsequent myocardial infarction. A closer examination of these symptoms suggested a roughly even division between features of anxiety and depression. In survivors of first myocardial infarction, around 55% of patients with psychological symptoms were anxious while 37% were depressed. Among patients experiencing a second or further myocardial infarction, around 42% reported anxiety, however 58% exhibited symptoms of overt depressive disorder (Cay et al., 1972). It has been suggested (Cay, Philip, & Aitken, 1976) that anxiety after myocardial infarction, if it is sufficiently long standing, can transform into symptoms of depression. The preponderance of depressive symptoms over those of anxiety in the sample of patients with second or subsequent myocardial infarctions might, therefore, reflect a continuation of emotional disturbance after the initial episode of illness, such that patients with a second episode are likely to be predisposed this time to the experience of depression. The time elapsing between first and second heart attack would clearly influence the logic of this reasoning. It is unfortunate then, that Cay et al. (1976) fail to expand on the time course over which anxiety is replaced by symptoms of depression.

The distinction between depression and anxiety in response to myocardial infarction is also reflected in results reported by Mayou et al. (1978). A study of 100 survivors of first myocardial infarction revealed that 32% complained of moderate symptoms of psychological distress; a further 32% complained of marked symptoms of distress within two months after the onset of illness. Of these patients, rather more than half reported either tension or situational anxiety, while something less than half were troubled by symptoms of depression. Moreover, depression would seem to be most evident later rather than soon in the process of recovery and rehabilitation after myocardial infarction (Segers & Mertens, 1975). Therefore while both anxiety and depression occur with notable frequency after myocardial infarction (Dreyfuss, Dasberg, & Assael, 1969; Cay et al., 1972; Mayou et al., 1978), the latter is most likely to be of clinical prominence in the later stages of the illness when the patient has had sufficient time to comprehend the reality of the threat to life and the potential for future incapacity (Degré-Coustry & Grevisse, 1982).

Anxiety, on the other hand, is probably the most common immediate emotional response to acute myocardial infarction (Groen, 1976) and this would seem to be consistent with a wealth of evidence on emotional responses to all serious physical illness (Lipowski, 1975). While this may metamorphose to a depressive state if severe and prolonged (Cay et al., 1976) or initiate denial among those predisposed to that defense mechanism (Soloff, 1978), there is little doubt that in the acute phase of myocardial infarction it is anxiety that is the predominant emotional response and, therefore, the most immediate focus for management.

A number of detailed studies have built on the observations of Cay et al. (1972). Psychometric scales of anxiety were administered to a sample of 286 men admitted to an intensive coronary-care unit with acute symptoms of myocardial infarction and these measures were subsequently given to the same patients four days, seven days 10 days, and four months after admission to hospital (Dellipiani, Cay, Philip, Vetter, Colling, Donaldson, & McCormick, 1976). In common with the earlier work of Cay and her group, the patients for this study were drawn from the area around Edinburgh. It was found that during the early stages of illness, levels of anxiety were high relative to normal population data. These, however, fell rapidly between the fourth and seventh days when most patients were transferred from the intensive coronary-care unit to a general medical ward. At this point, levels of anxiety in survivors of myocardial infarction were no greater than those for other parients with medical conditions in general wards. Anxiety levels rose again, however, as patients approached the end of their stay in hospital and contemplated the posthospital phase of their illness. At four months after admission to hospital, anxiety levels had once more fallen and were again equivalent to those found in the general population. The importance of these data are twofold. Firstly, levels of anxiety were objectively assessed using standard psychometric instruments rather than inferred from subjective psychiatric diagnoses. This confers the joint advantages of replicability and comparability with normative data. Secondly, measures of anxiety were taken serially over time so that the natural history of the emotional response could be gauged. In this respect, it is interesting to note that the fluctuations observed in anxiety levels over time seems consistent with the preceived seriousness of the challenge being faced by patients at particular points in the progress of their illness. Thus it is entirely sensible that anxiety should be high soon after symptom onset when life threat is greatest, and then again when patients are reminded that they must soon relinquish constant medical attention and face a possibly lengthy period of rehabilitation, but that anxiety should fall to normal or near-normal levels once more when patients are able to re-evaluate the threat of death or disability in the light of posthospital experience.

In a study of a similar group of patients drawn from the same geographical area (Vetter, Cay, Philip, & Strange, 1977), it was shown that levels of anxiety among patients admitted to an intensive coronary-care unit was no greater than that among patients admitted as medical emergencies to other hospital wards. Women showed higher levels of anxiety in response to myocardial infarction than men. Moreover patients with the less critical condition of myocardial ischemia (anginal pain) but with symptoms mimicking those of myocardial infarction, responded with greater levels of anxiety than patients who were aware they had sustained a myocardial infarction. One possible explanation for this hinges on the proposition that the certainty associated with an unequivocal diagnosis of myocardial infarction may actually limit experienced anxiety, whereas the relative uncertainty of a diagnosis of myocardial ischemia, with so many unanswered questions about the symptoms and their meanings, may enhance the fear associated with admission to intensive coronary care.

Wrzesniewski (1977) investigated levels of anxiety in a consecutive series of 105 male survivors of first myocardial infarction. Both specific anxiety (anxiety associated with the myocardial infarction) and general anxiety (anxiety as a generalized personality predisposition) were measured 15 days after the myocardial infarction. These data were compared with levels of anxiety in a group of healthy men free from coronary disease and in a group of patients with rheumatic disease who were attending at a general hospital for outpatient treatment. Both comparison groups were matched for occupational status with the sample of survivors of myocardial infarction. Both specific and general anxiety were significantly and quite markedly elevated in the patients with myocardial infarction relative to both comparison groups; however, this anxiety dissipated with time and was consonant with levels of anxiety in the comparison groups at around four months after admission to hospital. At both periods when anxiety was measured, there was a significant correlation between measures of specific and general anxiety, and this finding which emerged in later studies (Byrne, 1979) is of some importance in the clinical management of emotional reactions to myocardial infarction because it may allow the early detection of those who may go on to suffer protracted and undue emotional distress in response to illness.

A somewhat novel approach to the measurement of anxiety in patients in intensive coronary-care units was adopted by Froese, Cassem, Hackett, and Silverberg (1975). They measured electrodermal reactivity in a sample of 25 patients recovering from myocardial infarction, throughout the course of an interview that covered questions related to a broad range of issues and concerns since admission to hospital. In addition, standard psychometric scales of anxiety were administered at the time of psychophysiological testing. It was found that electrodermal reactivity as evidenced by the galvanic skin potential was a significant predictor of subjectively reported anxiety in these patients. Regrettably, no control subjects were examined and one can say little about levels of anxiety in these cardiac patients relative to patients with other illnesses or with no illness at all.

Byrne (1979) assessed both state anxiety (anxiety in response to the specific challenge of myocardial infarction) and trait anxiety (anxiety as a generalized response to environmental stressors) in a sample of 120 survivors of myocardial infarction and a comparison group of 40 patients admitted to a coronary-care unit with the appearance of myocardial infarction but discharged from that facility within 48 hours of admission with a confirmed diagnosis of some (less serious) illness. Some of these patients suffered chest pain of ischemic origin, some had pericarditis, and others had contracted pulmonary infections, though all were aware they had not sustained a heart attack. The two groups of patients were not differentiated by the measure of trait anxiety, indicating perhaps that both groups entered hospital with the same average tendency to respond to life crises with emotional distress. Measures of state anxiety did however differentiate between the two patient groups, with those suffering from myocardial infarction reporting higher levels of state anxiety than those for whom a lesser diagnosis was given. It was found, moreover, that measures of state and trait anxiety were significantly intercorrelated for both groups of patients. When patients with myocardial infarction were divided according to sex, it became evident that female patients exhibited generally higher levels of state anxiety than did male subjects, though this did not hold for measures of trait anxiety.

Segers and Mertens (1977a and 1977b) carried out a very detailed, qualitative examination of anxiety in samples of survivors of acute myocardial infarction, symptom-free subjects who had attended a screening clinic for the assessment of coronary risk factors and in whom such risk factors had in fact been detected and health volunteers in whom there was no evidence of cardiac disease or risk of it. Psychometric measures of anxiety failed to distinguish between the three groups, though this was attributed to higher standard deviations found for anxiety self-ratings of coronary patients. A closer investigation of patterns of anxiety for the three groups did, however, produce substantial distinctions which are worthy of note. Patients with myocardial infarction, though they appeared to be subject to ego-vulnerability and to disturbances of self-image were, however, able to manifest sufficient defence mechanisms such as obsessional self-control to cope with the stress of illness. Other subjects, by contrast, expressed rather more undifferentiated anxiety, perhaps related to the fact that they did not have a specific focus such as myocardial infarction upon which to attribute the cause of their distress. They did, however, also manifest a variety of psychopathological characteristics such as dependency, feelings of weakness and powerlessness, and a tendency to somatize, in contrast to the apparently more controlled behaviors of patients with myocardial infarction, though the distinctions may be due in part to the apparently urgent mobilization of defence mechanisms among patients with coronary disease.

The collective data on affective distress after myocardial infarction are not in complete agreement. The findings of Byrne (1979) that patients with myocardial infarction experienced higher levels of anxiety than those with a less serious medical diagnosis do not precisely accord with the results of Vetter et al. (1977) that patients with the uncertain diagnosis of myocardial ischemia were more highly anxious than patients with myocardial infarction. This disparity may, however, be best viewed in the light of the relative certainty or otherwise of diagnoses. In the former study, patients in the noninfarction group were sure that at worst they had received a warning of cardiac problems, while in the latter they appear to have been faced with a rather less definite explanation of their symptoms. This aside, the bulk of the literature supports the contention that anxiety, at least, is a characteristic accompaniment to the early phases of recovery from myocardial infarction.

Significant relationships between measures of state and trait anxiety have consistently emerged in the literature (Wrzesniewski, 1977; Byrne, 1979). These relationships give support to the more general suggestion of Cay et al. (1976) that those patients with a pre-existing neurotic disposition will respond with the greatest emotional disturbance to the crisis of myocardial infarction and are very much in accord with the notion that the intensity of an affective response to any challenge (state anxiety) is modulated by an individual predisposition to neuroticism (trait anxiety) (Speilberger, 1972).

The evidence is also clear that different kinds of people express anxiety in response to myocardial infarction in different ways and to different degrees. Women with myocardial infarction report greater state anxiety than do men (Vetter et al. 1977; Byrne, 1979) though this result cannot be explained in terms of a stronger neurotic predisposition to anxiety responses among these women patients (Byrne, 1979). This sex difference would seem to reflect a more generalized phenomenon related to sex differences in emotional behavior in response to the challenge of illness. Brown and Rawlinson (1977) found women to be more reluctant than men to relinquish the sick role following cardiac surgery. Sex differences too, were apparent in emotional responses to cancer (Haney,

1977), with women more likely than men to experience severe and protracted emotional distress, though this is clearly confounded by variations in the site of the cancer and whether it was associated with reproductive tissue. It may also be confounded by the relative effectiveness of denial and other defense mechanisms in male patients. The issue of sex differences in the presentation of emotional distress is a controversial one (Phillips & Segal, 1969; Byrne, 1981) and such differences in psychological responses to illness need to be interpreted with some caution. The fact that these appear in the absence of sex differences in predisposing neurotic traits does, however, indicate the finding to be a real rather than an apparent one.

Sociooccupational class, too, appears to influence emotional reactions to myocardial infarction, though the evidence is not consistent on the direction of this influence. Byrne (1981) found that blue-collar workers exhibited higher levels of state anxiety in response to myocardial infarction than did white-collar workers. Both Croog and Levine (1977) and Dominian and Dobson (1969) found persons of lower social class to experience more difficulties in hospital after myocardial infarction than persons of higher social class, the reasons for this relating either to faulty communications with their physicians or failure to interpret the hospital environment in a reassuring way. In reporting on similar findings, Hackett and Cassem (1976) suggested that patients of higher social class probably enjoyed a greater exchange of information with their physicians than did patients of lower social class—reflecting, presumably, the benefits of educational, social, and financial compatibility between higher-social-status patients and their physicicans. This finding may, however, also reflect a greater readiness by educated and articulate patients of higher social status to actively seek information from physicians and others regarding their cardiac conditions.

By contrast, Rosen and Bibring (1966) reported that persons of higher social class were more likely to respond to myocardial infarction with anxiety than persons of lower social class. They speculated that this was due to the more adequate use of denial among persons of lower social class. However, while the evidence is, once more, not clearcut, its general thrust supports the argument that those in lower socioeconomic groupoings are more likely to experience emotional distress after myocardial infarction than are those in higher socioeconomic groupings. These data give substance to Doehrman's (1977) claim that ". . .social factors such as social class and employment opportunities might be related to a patient's view of his life in hospital and his attitudes towards the future," and perhaps, therefore, to emotional responses to illness. Limited employment opportunities and a more uncertain occupational and social future for cardiac patients in lower socioeconomic groupings may in fact provide a set of social stressors to which anxiety and other emotional disturbance is a very realistic and reasonable response.

The clinical importance of emotional distress following myocardial infarction, and anxiety in particular, is now receiving considerable recognition (Vetter et al. 1977; Byrne, 1979). Mather, Pearson, and Read (1971) noted an increased mortality among patients with myocardial infarction who were treated in hospital relative to those who were treated at home (the two groups being presumably unselected for severity of infarction), and speculated that this might be due to the additional anxiety generated by the coronary-care-unit atmosphere. Indeed, this often-praised addition to modern medical treatment has been seen as a potential psychological hazard (Hackett, Cassem, & Wishnie, 1968) and there is an apparently increasing trend to offer psychological intervention early in the course of myocardial infarction to alleviate the specific anxiety generated by the coronary-care unit itself (Cay et al., 1976). There is a growing body of comment that the technology and setting of the coronary-care unit, necessary as these are, produce a range of subjective responses to the experience (Geersten, Ford, & Castle, 1976) and that anxiety and apprehension predominate among these responses. Lee and Ball (1975) were led to comment, "When a patient is totally dependent on strangers and mysterious machines, conditions are right for psychological trauma." There is some speculation then that at least part of the emotional distress occurring in the short term after myocardial infarction may be attributed to the experience of the intensive coronary-care unit.

Razin (1982), however, pointed out that there is by no means universal agreement with this view. For some patients at least, the medical environment and the presence of equipment for cardiac monitoring and resuscitation acted as a reassurance that medical care was rapidly available in case of complications, thus alleviating some of the anxiety associated with hospitalization. There is, in fact, now evidence that release from the coronary-care unit into a general medical ward and away from the environment of intensive medical scrutiny acts to increase anxiety in some patients (Klein, Kliner, Zipes, Troyer & Wallace, 1968) and may even enhance physiological vulnerability to cardiological complications unless the patient is suitably prepared for the experience.

The time course for emotional distress following myocardial infarction is extremely variable. Some patients will experience fear immediately on recognition of the symptoms of heart attack, leading in some instances to denial of the significance of these and a delay in seeking medical care (Surwit et al., 1982). For others the symptoms at onset will be of sufficient intensity for clouding or loss of consciousness to occur, so that any recognition of the real implications of the situation will be delayed until some days after admission to hospital. Others still will be able to mobilize denial sufficiently rapidly that emotional distress never becomes manifest, though while there is little doubt that denial is to be widely seen following myocardial infarction (Croog, Shapiro, & Levine, 1971) its real extent has been challenged (Soloff, 1978).

Many studies of emotional distress after heart attack have limited their enquiry to the period of hospitalization. It is important to recognize that the patient does not revert to normality immediately upon discharge but may continue to experience both anxiety and depression well into the period of recovery and rehabilitation.

Anxiety after myocardial infarction, from whatever source, insofar as it is associated with the liberation of sympathetic monoamines into the cardiovascular system (Frankenhaeuser, 1975), might certainly prove noxious to a myocardium that is still physiologically vulnerable some days after the onset of illness (Cole, McCall, Reader & Woodings, 1977). Moreover, there is experimental evidence (Volicer & Volicer, 1978) that increases in heart rate and both systolic and diastolic blood pressure are positively associated with subjective reports of distress during hospitalization for serious illness. The physiological conditions whereby anxiety following myocardial infarction could precipitate cardiac complications, particularly in a vulnerable patient, seem therefore to be established.

There is little doubt that anxiety is elevated in survivors of myocardial infarction at some time during recovery, both in response to the illness itself, with its myriad of personal and psychosocial implications for the individual patient, and in response to the unfamiliar technical atmosphere of the modern coronary-care unit. The evidence would indicate that at least part of the intensity of this anxiety may be explained in terms of a predisposing neurotic trait toward anxiety in the face of crisis. If early psychological intervention is to be used most effectively to alleviate this potentially noxious anxiety, it would be well for those charged with the care of patients with myocardial infarction to know at the point of admission to coronary care which patients are most likely to exhibit manifest anxiety of clinical proportions at some stage during their recovery. This may involve, among other things, the collection of information by interview from close relatives concerning the ways in which the patient may have responded to previous life crises or coped with difficulties in the past. Such an exercise would have the effect of sensitizing medical staff in coronary-care units to those patients likely to be at risk with respect to intense anxiety after myocardial infarction and to facilitate the use of psychological intervention services to coronary-care units at a point where this may be most indicated.

3.   ILLNESS BEHAVIOR AS A GLOBAL RESPONSE TO MYOCARDIAL INFARCTION

Symptoms of emotional distress represent one clearcut dimension of psychological responses to myocardial infarction. It is now clear, however, that a much more diverse range of behaviors is elicited by the challenge of this illness, and this collection of responses distinguishes not only between patients with myocardial infarction and patients with other serious illness, but also varies widely between individual survivors of myocardial infarction. This diversity of reactions may be discussed under the general umbrella of illness behavior. While there have been a variety of clinical and sociological definitions of illness behavior, it is generally taken to refer to the collective responses—whether cognitive, affective, or behavioral—which any individual has to the personal challenge of serious illness (Lipowski, 1975).

Studies directed toward the description of the totality of responses to myocardial infarction have been rather sparse. Wrzesniewski (1980) developed a scale to measure attitudes toward illness in patients who had experienced a myocardial infarction. Administration of this scale to a sample of survivors of myocardial infarction and subsequent multivariate analysis of the data yielded six characteristic sets of attitudes to the illness. These represented the degree of anxiety associated with the present experience of myocardial infarction, the current mood state, the intensity of the patient's demands for care, the patient's perceptions of future activity after illness, the degree of acceptance of the diagnosis and medical recommendations which had been made for recovery, and the extent and adequacy of information the patient perceived he was given regarding both the illness and its treatment. These sets of attitudes were found to be quite strongly intercorrelated and were refined into a single scale, the extremes of which defined highly positive and highly negative attitudes toward myocardial infarction. It was found that the more neurotic the patient (as identified by scores on the neuroticism scale of the Eysenck Personality Inventory), the more negative the attitudes to myocardial infarction were likely to be. This tendency was paralleled for measures of state anxiety, where high levels of situational anxiety as identified by scores on both the Taylor Manifest Anxiety Scale and on the State scale of the Speilberger State Trait Anxiety Inventory also correlated with negative attitudes toward myocardial infarction. The strong intercorrelations between the several attitude scales described by Wrzesniewski (1980) do not, however, allow a complete account of the range of responses to myocardial infarction which would be expected from anecdotal reports.

The clinical implications of illness behavior for recovery and rehabilitation following myocardial infarction prompted a series of studies by Byrne and Whyte (1978). These studies were based on the notion that individuals will adopt characteristic patterns of perceiving, evaluating, and reacting in relation to their illnesses (Mechanic, 1966); and should these responses be inappropriate to the nature of the illness (Pilowsky, 1969), it may be exacerbated or its course prolonged (Wrzesniewski, 1975). The idea that inappropriate responses to illness can influence the course of recovery from that illness has its theoretical basis in the concept of ''abnormal illness behavior'' (Pilowsky, 1969) and should be conceptually distinguished from illness behavior as help-seeking behavior following the onset of symptoms (Mechanic, 1966). This latter notion is, of course, relevant to the actions patients might take in the early and critical pre-hospital phase of their illness. Two distinct studies of illness behaviour, one with patients reporting intractable pain (Pilowsky & Spence, 1975), and the other on long-term haemodialysis patients (Pritchard, 1977), have shown sufficiently disparate results to suggest that patterns of illness behaviour are strongly influenced by the nature of the illness.

The clinical importance of the work of Byrne and Whyte (1978) lies in the comprehensive account of illness behavior following myocardial infarction. Patients making up the sample consisted of survivors of myocardial infarction aged 35 to 65 years (mean age = 52.4) admitted to coronary-care units in a medium-sized city over the course of a 12-month sampling period. These patients had all attracted an unequivocal diagnosis of myocardial infarction as defined by serial EKG changes, elevated serum enzymes, and a typical clinical history of chest pain (see Chapter 1). The sample was, as far as possible, a consecutive series of patients with myocardial infarction admitted to intensive coronary care during the sampling period.

Assessment of illness behavior evident among patients in the sample was made using a questionnaire developed and reported by Pilowsky and Spence (1975). This was a 62 item self-report instrument constructed to assess ". . .the patient's attitudes and feelings about his illness, his perceptions of the reactions of significant others in the environment (including his doctors) to himself and to his illness, and the patient's own view of his current psychosocial condition." It has been used to gather data in a wide variety of clinical settings and Pilowsky and Spence (1975) have suggested it to be broadly relevant to the assessment of responses to illness in many clinical groups. The instrument was introduced to each patient as a means of ". . .asking you about your own reactions to being ill and to being in hospital." It was administered in a general medical ward following the patient's discharge from intensive coronary care between 10 and 14 days after admission to hospital. All patients were aware they had sustained a myocardial infarction and had freely consented to being interviewed.

A factor analysis of patients' responses revealed eight orthogonal factors accounting for 61.5% of the variance each of which conveyed clinical meaning within the context of a wealth of past material, albeit anecdotal, on the range of responses which patients might make to the experience of myocardial infarction. These were:

a. Factor I (19.9% variance) characterized by items reflecting general somatic concern and a single item suggesting concern with psychological functioning. Principal factor loadings were on items relating to one's own and other people's states of health and one's own appearance. Pilowsky and Spence (1975) obtained a general factor defined by a similar conglomerate of items and labeled it "Hypochondriasis." However, as the main focus of this factor seems to center on both health and appearance, it seems more appropriate to label it *somatic concern*.

b. Factor II (8.7% of variance) characterized by items relating to the recognition that personal, social, and financial worries prior to illness may have contributed to the present episode of myocardial infarction, and labeled *psychosocial precipitants*.

c. Factor III (7.1% of variance) characterized by items suggesting an affective response to illness to the point where interpersonal relationships are interfered with and labeled affective *disruption*.

d. Factor IV (6.0% of variance) characterized by items indicating difficulty in expressing personal feelings, and labeled *affective inhibition*.

e. Factor V (5.8% of variance) characterized by items indicating a recognition by the patient of the presence of serious illness, and labeled *illness recognition*.

f. Factor VI (5.4% of variance) characterized by items suggesting the experience of subjective tension, and labeled *subjective tension*.

g. Factor VII (4.4% of variance) characterized by items indicating a recognition and acceptance of the sick role, and labeled *sick-role acceptance*.

h. Factor VIII (4.2% of variance) characterized by items suggesting acceptance of medical reassurance, and labeled *trust in the doctor*.

The items defining these factors together with the factor loadings are presented in Table 3.1, which follows.

While reporting on a factor-analytic study is essentially an exercise in clinical interpretation, emergent patterns of intercorrelated results are often both theoretically sensible and of clinical utility. Dimensions of illness behavior should relate to the affective, behavioral, and cognitive meanings that a particular illness holds for those afflicted with it (Lipowski, 1975). To allow confidence in their veracity, they should also be consistent with prevailing attitudes and views, gleaned from both clinical and empirical sources, on how individuals should be expected to respond to a given illness with its own particular characteristics. Factors emerging from this study were indeed both appropriate and relevant to common preconceptions of the experience of myocardial infarction.

Concern for one's state of health, sometimes of hypochondriacal proportions, has been a prominent finding in many studies of illness behavior (Pilowsky, 1967; Pilowsky & Spence, 1975). The first and largest factor emerging from the study of Byrne and Whyte (1978) was defined by items distinctly germane to this concern. Collectively, they depicted an attitude of concern and, in the extreme, a preoccupation with bodily function and dysfunction extending to concern with appearance and psychological function. Certainly, patients affirming these items may have done so prior to illness. However, such attributes have not been found to characterize potential sufferers of myocardial infarction (Ostfeld, Lebovits, & Shekelle, 1964) but become evident only after the experience of the clinical event (Lebovits, Shekelle, & Ostfeld, 1967). Enhanced sensitivity to one's somatic state and a concern for its correct functioning would, therefore, appear to be mobilized by the experience of myocardial infarction.

Table 3.1. Factors Reflecting Self-Descriptions of Illness Behavior Following First Survived Myocardial Infarction

Illness Behavior Attributes	Factor Loadings
Factor I	
Jealous of other people's good health	+0.76
Sensitized to illness fear through publicity	+0.72
Thinks something the matter with mind	+0.55
Upset by appearance of face or body	+0.49
Believes more liable to illness than others	+0.46
More sensitive to pain than others	+0.45
Factor II	
Problems in life other than illness	+0.75
Personal worries not caused by illness	+0.74
Family problems	+0.56
Financial problems	+0.50
Work problems	+0.46
Believes symptoms caused by worry	+0.42
Factor III	
Gets anxious easily	+0.69
Gets sad easily	+0.60
Illness influences relationships with others	+0.41
Factor IV	
Hard to show personal feelings	+0.77
Can express personal feelings to others	−0.71
Factor V	
Illness interfers with life patterns	+0.68
Thinks something seriously wrong with body	+0.62
Worries about possibility of serious illness	+0.59
Factor VI	
Has trouble with nerves	+0.68
Finds it hard to relax	+0.59
Often gets depressed	+0.45
Factor VII	
Obsessional thoughts about health	+0.69
Annoyed when reassured by others	+0.54
Frequently tries to explain to others how feeling	+0.43
Factor VIII	
Easily cheered up by doctor	+0.59
Expresses belief in doctor's judgment	+0.41

The second aspect of illness behavior, that which was labeled psychosocial precipitants, appeared to be a corroboration from the patient's viewpoint of the well-documented notion that clinical episodes of myocardial infarction are commonly preceded by an accumulation of worrying or distressing life circumstances (Byrne & Whyte, 1980). The items defining the factors suggested, firstly, the recognition that worrying circumstances existed prior to myocardial infarction and, secondly, the realization that these may have contributed to the present illness.

Emotional or affective responses to illness are commonly observed forms of illness behavior (Lipowski, 1970; Pilowsky & Spence 1975; Pritchard 1977). Two qualitatively unique factors emerged from the study of Byrne and Whyte (1978) to represent this. The first of these, labeled affective disruption, suggested an affective response to illness to the point where interpersonal relationships were disrupted. While affective responses to illness are quite common, the disruptive effect of these has not previously been described in relation to patients with myocardial infarction. It may however resemble the irritability previously reported in relation to patients with intractable pain (Pilowsky & Spence, 1975). The second of these "affective" factors, that labeled subjective tension, carried with it a quality of psychological distress and agitation. Patients identifying with this aspect of illness behaviour felt an inability to relax and were continually troubled by nervous apprehension. Such tension could well be seen to have been mobilized by the illness, however, as there is some evidence, albeit of variable quality, that states of anxiety and tension precede myocardial infarction, one cannot exclude the possibility that this behavior reflects a pre-morbid attribute of the patient.

The factor labeled affective inhibition, which deals with the inability to express affect in response to myocardial infarction, is identical to a factor described by Pilowsky and Spence (1975) in relation to patients with intractable pain. Insofar as this relates to behavior mobilized by myocardial infarction, it may compare with an attribute of obsessional control of affect reported by Segers and Mertens (1977) in patients with coronary heart disease. This may, however, also reflect the operation of denial which has been found to be a common response in some survivors of myocardial infarction (Soloff, 1978) and which will be discussed later.

One single factor represented the patient's recognition that they were suffering from a serious illness. The emergence of this factor, labeled illness recognition, is not at all surprising, because all patients in this study were aware that they had sustained a myocardial infarction. Of course, not all patients affirmed items defining this factor, so that while they had most definitely suffered a myocardial infarction, they were either reluctant to admit to this or were concerned to de-emphasize its impact on their present or future lives. This may reflect the operation, among some patients, of denial of sufficient strength to override the recognition of a medically substantiated fact. Thematically related to illness recognition was the factor labeled sick-role acceptance. Items on this factor represented an affirmation of the sick role (Parsons, 1951) and a wish that this be accepted by significant others. In at least a subgroup of survivors of myocardial infarction, then, there would appear to be not only the realization of the presence of serious illness, but also the perhaps coexistent recognition of the particular social role this endows them with. The final factor reported by Byrne and Whyte (1978), that labeled trust in the doctor, clearly reflected a response mobilized by the experiences of myocardial infarction. This expression of confidence in the medical attention being received was a positive attribute and has previously been observed in survivors of myocardial infarction (Cay et al., 1972; Wrzesniewski, 1975), though it may be evident from the earlier discussion of anxiety following heart attack that the absence of such confidence can lead to considerable emotional distress.

These results in comparison with data from other work suggest that patterns of illness behavior following myocardial infarction are substantially different from those following other illnesses. Illness behavior, as we have noted, is an expression of the affective behavioral and cognitive meanings a particular illness has for those afflicted with it. It can be seen to arise from the interplay between the nature of the illness and the psychological characteristics of the individual. Because illnesses vary in terms of severity, chronicity, the amount of information avilable to the patient, the expected prognosis, the subjective perception of the physiological state, the degree of experienced pain and discomfort, and many other factors, it is not surprising that an illness as potentially dramatic in presentation and cause as myocardial infarction elicits such a characteristic pattern of emotional and behavioral responses. The factors emerging from the study of Byrne and Whyte (1978), and particularly those involving heightcncd somatic concern, anxiety, and depression, recognition of the presence of serious illness, acceptance of the sick role, and explicit trust in the doctor, are all consistent with an illness which presents an acute clinical episode, sometimes dramatic in onset, potentially life endangering, and portentous of residual disability. These factors are very much in agreement with the diversity of responses to myocardial infarction previously observed and documented in the literature (Vetter, Cay, Philip, & Strange, 1977; Wrzesniewski, 1975; Cay et al., 1972).

Three issues are, however, of ongoing importance in assessing the significance of behavior following myocardial infarction. Firstly, there is the issue of whether patterns of illness behavior are consistent across individuals after myocardial infarction or whether illness behavior reflects wide individual variation in actions and affects. Secondly, if such diversity is apparent, the characteristics of the illness, the individual, and the environment as determining influences come into question. Finally, and most important clinically, is the issue of whether patterns of illness behavior after myocardial infarction are in any way predictive of recovery and rehabilitation, for it is in this issue that the ultimate utility of the measurement of illness behavior lies.

While the experience of myocardial infarction imparts an identifiable character to illness behavior issuing from it, any overview of the literature on responses to this illness reflects a fundamental diversity between individuals in the ways they perceive, feel, and act in the face of such a challenge. The theoretical literature on illness behavior does, in fact, make a fundamental distinction between the normal and abnormal forms of the phenomenon. The former refers to patterns of behavior, affect, and thought which are adaptive and expected within the context of a life-threatening illness. The latter (Pilowsky, 1969) deals with responses which are out of context to the precipitating situation and which, if prolonged, might interfere with the course of recovery and rehabilitation after illness. Such aspects of abnormal illness behavior might vary from undue and excessive emotional responses through to a failure to comply with medical instructions; however, their common feature is that of maladaptability and of incompatibility with a normal recovery.

The diversity of illness behavior following myocardial infarction remains to be fully explored. Byrne, Whyte, and Lance (1979) attempted to examine this by using a cluster analytic technique. Such analyses establish logical classifications by dividing a heterogeneous group of individuals into smaller and more homogeneous subgroups on the basis of commonly held attribute profiles, so exploiting the variation in illness behavior within a single sample of patients. While a review of the mathematics of cluster analysis would not add appreciably to the present discussion, this has been closely examined in material dealing with the logic of classification (Everitt, 1974; Hartigan, 1976). A range of cluster analytic procedures are available for use; however the work of Byrne et al. (1978) employed a divisive polythetic algorithm devised by Lance and Williams (1975). Data for this classificatory process consisted of factor scores for the eight illness behavior dimensions described by Byrne and Whyte (1978) taken from the same sample of survivors of myocardial infarction used to derive the factors.

This process yielded thematically distinct and mutually exclusive clusters of patients, with each being made up of patients having common profiles of illness-behavior attributes. Patients in the first cluster exhibited significantly higher factor scores than those of the rest of the sample for all illness behavior factors but that representing trust in the doctor. It suggests a group of patients whose experience of myocardial infarction enhanced their somatic awareness, triggered depression and anxiety with concomitant disruption of interpersonal relationships, allowed a recognition of the presence of a serious illness and an acceptance of the sick role and precipitated a prevailing state of subjectively felt affective distress. The most obvious interpretation of this pattern of attributes is that patients holding these are responding to an indisputably serious illness by emphasizing that it has been an event of considerable impact and wide-ranging consequence in their lives.

The second cluster consisted of a group of patients expressing significantly higher levels of affective disruption, illness recognition, and sick-role acceptance than patients in the remainder of the sample. The cluster would appear to be composed of a group of patients expressing a realistic recognition and acceptance of the presence of illness and the social role it endows them with but who nonetheless are distressed by the illness and its interpersonal consequences.

Patients composing the third cluster exhibited significantly higher scores on the illness behavior dimensions of illness recognition, subjective tension, and sick-role acceptance than those in the rest of the sample. This is not unlike the pattern of illness acceptance exhibited by patients in the second cluster, though the emotional consequences do not appear to be evident to the same degree.

The final cluster, to which by far the greatest number of patients held membership, was characterized by cluster mean scores which were lower than sample mean scores for all of the defining illness behavior attributes. This suggests a group of patients expressing the attitude that their illness is of little consequence to them, having only a weak emotional impact, with the tendency even to deemphasize recognition of the presence of the illness itself.

The emergence of four clusters of patients, with each cluster exhibiting a qualitatively unique representation of the eight demensions of illness behavior upon which the cluster analysis was based, reflects the presence of considerable individual variation in responses to myocardial infarction. The first of the clusters represents probably the most pronounced form of illness behavior to be seen in survivors of myocardial infarction and would suggest that the experience of illness for patients within this cluster has been one of profound impact. Patients composing this cluster were not only prepared to recognize the existence of their illness and accept the role it endowed them with but were also considerably troubled by the event, expressing depression, anxiety, and concern with their level of physiological integrity. One is hesitant to claim this as an excessive response to myocardial infarction, as the illness itself is undeniably dramatic and serious, and an attitude of strong concern may be altogether realistic. However, it is not uncommon for such concern to become preoccupation with bodily function and debilitating anxiety and depression (Cay et al., 1976).

The second cluster was clearly defined by fewer aspects of illness behavior than the first, these aspects representing an acceptance of illness and an affective response to it. The fact that both illness recognition and sick-role acceptance were represented in the cluster may indicate that the emotional distress also experienced by this group of patients occurs in response not only to the presence of a life-threatening illness but also to the danger that it may enforce on them an uncharacteristic social role. The sick role, with its implications of prolonged disability and deviance is certainly reported to be a source of concern for some survivors of myocardial infarction (Finlayson & McEwen, 1977). The third cluster was not unlike the second, except that the degree of emotional distress experienced appeared to be of a less intense nature than that represented in the second cluster. It is possible that this cluster, with the minimum intrusion of emotional distress, represents the most realistic and rational approach to illness of all of the clusters of illness behavior emerging from the analysis.

The final cluster was almost indisputably one of denial, both of illness and its consequences. Patients composing this cluster would appear to have been both minimizing the seriousness of their myocardial infarction and claiming it to be of little continuing consequence in their lives. It is not surprising that such a large cluster emerged, because denial is a frequently described characteristic of survivors of myocardial infarction (Olin & Hackett, 1964; Froese et al., 1975; Levine & Ziegler, 1975; Soloff, 1977).

The application of Pilowsky's (1969) criteria for abnormal illness behavior that these should be responses out of proportion to the severity of the pathology and persistent in spite of reasonable medical reassurance is a difficult exercise with regard to myocardial infarction, for the pathology associated with this illness is undoubtedly severe and the residual cardiac incapacity may be long lasting. An additional criterion for abnormal illness behavior might be that it consists of a set of psychological responses to illness which are either themselves detrimental to the processes of recovery and rehabilitation or can be expected to produce physiological effects which might impede these processes. In this sense, some components of the several clusters already described can be viewed within the context of abnormal illness behavior. Wrzesniewski (1975) stated that attitudes most favoring the treatment and rehabilitation processes after myocardial infarction are characterized by ''. . .low level of fear connected with the fact of myocardial infarction, high level of acceptance of the diagnosis and medical recommendations and an even tempered mood.'' Only patients in the third cluster were characterized by these features, and it would appear that these patients coped with their illness most adequately of all. Patients occupying both the first and second clusters were identified not only by a recognition of the presence of illness but also by an expression of a marked emotional response to the event. In addition, patients in the first cluster appeared to emphasize the wide-ranging impact of myocardial infarction on their life-styles. Finlayson and McEwen (1977) noted this attitude among some survivors of myocardial infarction and found it to be related to an unwillingness to resume an active and productive life-style and an overdependence on the spouse or other family members, with a reciprocal overprotective attitude on the part of significant others. This is not dissimilar to care-eliciting behavior described by Henderson (1974), and insofar as it leads to prolonged and usually unnecessary invalidism, it may be considered abnormal illness behavior.

In a more specific sense, responses to illness involving unduly intense emotional distress might be considered detrimental to the processes of recovery and rehabilitation in at least two ways. Firstly, anxiety in particular has biochemical concomitants that would certainly be noxious to a vulnerable myocardium in the first few days after myocardial infarction (Frankenhaeuser, 1976). The comprehensive review of both human and animal studies (Lown, De Silva, Reich, & Murawski, 1980) has linked the liberation of catecholamines secondary to emotional distress with a range of potentially fatal cardiac amlythmias. Secondly, any emotional response, either anxiety or depression, if sufficiently long lasting, becomes pathological in itself (Cay et al., 1976) and imposes an additional illness load that can not help but impede recovery and rehabilitation.

The use of the defense mechanism of denial, as would appear to have occurred among patients in the fourth cluster, is common in the face of threat (Soloff, 1978). In the short term, it might exert a protective influence in that pronounced emotional responses to illness observed among patients in the first instance have contributed to myocardial infarction.

At least three of the clusters of patients surviving myocardial infarction described previously would, therefore, appear to have shown psychological responses to illness reflecting elements of abnormal illness behavior. Some of these—for example denial—may be maladative only at certain stages of the processes of recovery and rehabilitation. It can be argued, however, that patients showing abnormal illness behavior in any of its forms run an increased risk of a troubled recovery and a protracted if not incomplete rehabilitation.

The determinants of illness behavior, as with any other behavior, are unlikely to be simple. Since the concept encompasses the whole range of responses to myocardial infarction—cognitive, emotional, and behavior—one must look to a broad set of influences extending from the clear-cut (age, sex, and the like) to the more theoretically involved (past patterns of learning and individual patterns of personality). In each of these areas there is, regrettably, only the barest evidence from which to draw inferences on why a particular individual should respond to the challenge of myocardial infarction in particular ways.

The sex of the patient would appear to make little difference to patterns of ilness behavior observed after myocardial infarction. Female patients did express higher levels than males on the illness behavior factors described by Byrne and Whyte (1978) as indicating trust in the medical care being received and subjectively experienced tension. It was also apparent that women expressed greater state (but not trait) anxiety in response to illness than did men (Byrne, 1979). With particular regard to myocardial infarction, however, there was no general support for the notion that gender or sex-role stereotypes endow a distinctive quality to the ways in which patients respond to heart attack. This is in contrast to literature in other areas of illness where, for example, female responses to the challenge of cancer (Haney, 1977) or major cardiac surgery (Brown & Rawlinson, 1977) appeared more pronounced than for men. Several reasons might be advanced to account for this. Firstly, since myocardial infarction is traditionally thought of as a condition afflicting mainly men, though the epidemiological literature is now challenging this (Johnson, 1977), few studies of responses to heart attack have actually included women in their samples. Secondly, while state anxiety appears to be greater in women than in men after myocardial infarction, the evidence would suggest that women typically express higher levels of affect in response to threat than do men (Byrne, 1981), and the differences observed for myocardial infarction are more of general than particular importance. Finally, while there is growing speculation on the potential for sex-role socialization to influence both the causes and consequences of illness (Levi, 1978), the evidence remains contentious. It must then be concluded, for the present, that the sex of the patient plays little part in the shaping of responses to myocardial infarction.

More traditional views would, perhaps, have it that since women are not typically in the role of the breadwinner, the occurrence of myocardial infarction, with its threat of protracted disability, should elicit a more attenuated response in women than in men. The present-day emphasis on the entry of women into the work force and the changes which this brings to traditional sex roles (Levi, 1978) makes this view somewhat antiquated; any influence on illness behavior that might once have been attributed to gender is now more likely to be irrecoverably confounded by occupational status.

The evidence on occupation as an influence on illness behavior is, unfortunately, contentious and contradictory. Occupation and anxiety have been discussed earlier but with few clear-cut conclusions. While patients in lower occupational strata seem to respond to myocardial infarction with greater state anxiety than those higher on the scale, other forms of response seem little influenced by occupation. In this respect the most concerted investigation has been that of Croog and Levine (1977). Soon after hospitalization, white-collar workers were attributing the cause of their illness to work stress in greater proportions than blue-collar workers while, by contrast, blue-collar workers appeared to center on the physical demands of the job as contributing to their heart attacks. Those in blue-collar occupations certainly appeared to experience greater difficulty in returning to active employment after recovery, complicated often by discrepancies between their own perceptions of their health status and that of their employers (Croog & Levine, 1977). There is no evidence, however, that this influenced the ways in which patients chose to act in response to myocardial infarction.

The patient's level of education might be expected to influence the ways in which they respond to illness, since those with the demonstrated ability to assimilate and organize information should utilize these skills to take information regarding their own illness and adopt rational postures toward this based on an intelligent assessment of the evidence. This reasoning is incorporated into Hackett and Cassem's (1976) interpretation of the finding that patients in lower social classes respond to myocardial infarction with more emotional distress than patients high on the social strata. Neither this finding nor the interpretation of it is, however, universally accepted, and there is little evidence of a more generalized effect on education on illness behavior after heart attack.

The clinical importance of such influences, if they exist, lies with the possibility that approaches to intervention might not be broadly appropriate to all patients after myocardial infarction. A distinct effect of education, occupation, or sex on responses to illness may necessitate the use of separate intervention strategies for different kinds of patients. In view of the evidence that no such distinctions are apparent, the issue of the composition of intervention groups or the application of intervention strategies becomes somewhat simpler, though this must be the substance of another chapter.

While demographic characteristics appear to have little to do with responses to myocardial infarction, the matter of pre-morbid personality does. Evidence from both anecdotal works (Cay et al., 1966) and empirical studies (Wrzesniewski, 1975, 1977; Byrne & Whyte, 1983) suggest that possession of the pre-morbid attribute of trait anxiety or neuroticism predisposes to the experience of state anxiety in response to myocardial infarction. In addition to this, it has been shown that measures of more global responses to myocardial infarction are quite strongly related to neuroticism (Byrne & Whyte, 1983). These include the tendency for the patient's emotional state to disrupt personal and social relationships and the readiness with which the patient takes up and maintains the sick role. Data such as these indicate quite clearly that illness behavior following myocardial infarction can not be attributed entirely to the nature of the illness, the setting in which it occurs, or the simple, demographic descriptors applying to the individual patient. It would also appear to be dependent on the ways in which the individual is motivated to organize behavior in general and respond to crises in particular. The real importance of this, as some (for example Mayou, 1984) have foreshadowed, is that it may be possible very soon after the patient's hospitalization with myocardial infarction to predict, on the basis of existing personality, whether a particular individual is likely to cope adequately with the challenge of illness or whether a response of emotional crisis might be expected. This prior warning has clear implications for the behavioral management of the cardiac patient even in the early stages of the illness.

4.   OVERVIEW

Psychological responses to myocardial infarction cover a broad range of manifestations within the realms of emotion and behavior. It is clear that these responses are characterized by considerable diversity, so that the illness behavior shown by one individual is unlikely to be an exact replica of that shown by any other. These individual differences have been both described and explored by multivariate techniques. It is also clear that the determinants of illness behavior are not simple but involve considerations ranging from the nature of the illness to the personality of the victim.

The clinical utility of the concern with illness behavior following myocardial infarction rests, however, with the relationship this has with outcome following the illness. The demonstration that particular patterns of illness behavior predispose to particular implications for the management of the survivor of myocardial infarction suggests that outcome could be altered by the process of behavior modification. The following chapter considers determinants of outcome after heart attack and looks in detail at the role illness behavior plays in this process.

CHAPTER 4

Determinants of Outcome Following Coronary Heart Disease

1. THE COURSE OF RECOVERY AND REHABILITATION

The range of potential outcomes awaiting the survivor of myocardial infarction, together with the literature documenting the relative distribution of such people to categories of outcomes, have been outlined in the previous chapters. It is clear that outcome after myocardial infarction can no longer be considered as a univariate concept. While such clear-cut end points as subsequent mortality, morbidity, and return to work offer a convenient focus of attention for epidemiologists, the more-difficult-to-measure outcomes of emotional and social disability cannot be disregarded, because they form, collectively, the most frequent source of potential difficulty for the survivor of myocardial infarction. Moreover, it will also be evident from the previous chapters that the whole range of outcomes following myocardial infarction may not be readily apparent at any single point in time. Rather, the several aspects of outcome may emerge over a period of up to four years following the initial illness (Finlayson & McEwen, 1977), with cardiological complications predominating in the earlier stages of recovery, and occupational, emotional, and social disability remaining unrecognized until well into the period of rehabilitation.

Outcomes following myocardial infarction are not chance events but are determined by a broad range of factors that are, at least in principle, identifiable and measurable. Thus, while the certain prediction of particular outcomes for particular individuals is not possible, the medical pronouncement of individual prognoses is both scientifically feasible and has become routine clinical practice. Factors taken into account in the formulation of this prognosis range broadly from those that objectively identify and describe the compromised integrity of the patient's cardiovascular system (Humphries, 1977), through those that rest with information on the patients' demographic and social characteristics, to those requiring more subjective judgments. The precision with which these factors contribute to prognostic formulations is also a matter of some variability, with objective medical data being generally conceded as more useful in this respect than data deriving from clinical judgments of the patient's psychosocial condition. Recent evidence (Mayou et al., 1978b; Mayou, 1984; Philip, Cay, Stuckey, & Vetter, 1981) does, however, point to the potential importance of factors other than those reflecting the integrity of the cardiovascular system in determining outcome after myocardial infarction, and cautions against the premature discarding of social and emotional influences in the prediction of outcome. It is clear, therefore, that the determinants of outcome following myocardial infarction are multivariate, and it is likely that they interact in complex ways.

Within the context of the present book the relevance of a discussion on the determinants of outcome lies largely with the need to establish appropriate foci for intervention. In view of the complex determinants of outcomes, however, medical as well as psychosocial influences on recovery and rehabilitation must be jointly considered. Wherever appropriate, it is intended to relate each class of determinant both to the nature of the outcome measure, whether it be cardiological, occupational, or psychosocial, and to the period of recovery or rehabilitation at which the outcome measure is assessed.

2. ACUTE CARDIAC DYSFUNCTION AND THE MEDICAL PROGNOSTIC INDICATORS

Outcome in the first hours and days after myocardial infarction is almost exclusively determined by physiological factors. The primary cause of death at this stage appears to be the occurrence of ventricular arrhythmias (Willerson et al., 1982), and while continuous electrocardiographic (EKG) monitoring in the coronary-care unit has resulted in notable reductions in mortality from such arrhythmias (Rose, 1975), the overall death rate from cardiac complications of those who have survived myocardial infarction long enough to be admitted to a coronary-care unit, depending on the population under investigation, is still considerable.

Both the location and the clinical severity of the myocardial infarction bear on outcome. According to Willerson et al. (1982), patients with anterior infarctions have a higher mortality rate than patients with inferior infarctions—presumably because of the greater loss of left ventricular muscle in the former. Mortality in the first days after myocardial infarction is also higher for patients with transmural infarctions than for patients with nontransmural infarctions by a ratio of around 2.3:1 (Marmor et al., 1982). These authors also noted that early recurrent myocardial infarction during hospitalization has a markedly deleterious effect on survival, though this would be seen as self-evident by most cardiologists.

The extent of the myocardial infarction is also an important determinant of outcome (Willerson et al., 1982). Irreversible damage to more than 40% of the left ventricular muscle leads to a high expectation of cardiological complications, including cardiogenic shock, congestive heart failure, and ventricular arrhythmias and, therefore, to a higher risk of mortality. Patients with small infarctions are less likely to experience such complications; however, this seems dependent on the location of the infarction, and Willerson et al. (1982) suggest that strategically located, small infarctions, or multiple small infarctions, may result in complications as significant as a single large infarction.

Willerson et al. (1982) listed a series of life-threatening complications of acute myocardial infarction which have been shown to occur during hospitalization, either in a coronary-care unit or general medical ward. The most potent of these would seem to involve disturbances of the heart rhythm or of the conduction system regulating that rhythm. However, contributors to short-term mortality also include a loss to hemodynamic efficiency secondary to low systolic arterial blood pressure and an impaired average cardiac output index. The influence of blood pressure on short-term survival rates has also been noted (Humphries, 1977) with both hypotension associated with cardiogenic shock and acute systolic hypertension on admission to coronary-care units being implicated in decreased survival rates, both in and following hospitalization.

Prospective investigation of outcome after myocardial infarction has sought empirical substantiation for a range of cardiological factors contributing to this process. These studies have typically concerned themselves either with the late hospital phase or post hospital phase of outcome following myocardial infarction. Christensen, Ford, Reading, and Castle (1977) compared the characteristics of 47 patients who died suddenly during the late hospital phase of acute myocardial infarction with those of a consecutive series of surviving patients sampled over the same time period. Risk factors which were significantly associated with sudden death during the late hospital phase involved prior cardiovascular disease, circulatory failure while in the coronary care unit, and documented arrhythmias and conduction disturbances, also during coronary-care admission. The relative risk for patients exhibiting all three of these risk factors was 6.0 in relation to patients with no risk factors at all, and relative risk appeared to be uniformly greater for male than female patients. Multiple risk factors were associated with a greater risk than were single risk factors.

In a prospective study of 200 consecutive patients with myocardial infarction, Marmor et al. (1981) investigated 14 clinical variables ranging from precoronary risk factors to complications documented during the coronary-care admission in an attempt to identify the determinants of early (in hospital) recurrent myocardial infarction. A multiple logistic regression analysis indicated three variables, those of preinfarction obesity, female sex, and recurrent chest pain during hospitalization, to be statistically associated with recurrent infarction during hospitalization.

In a further study to assess the power of these variables to predict recurrent myocardial infarction in the longer term, a consecutive series of 150 new patients were followed prospectively over an average of nine months following release from hospital (Marmor et al., 1982). Regression coefficients derived from the multiple logistic analysis of the initial sample (200 patients) and weighted on the three factors mentioned above, were able to predict short-term recurrent infarction in 80% of the subsequent sample (150 patients). Life table analysis performed to assess the influence of clinical factors on longer-term survival also identified continuing lipid disorder (elevated serum cholesterol or elevated serum triglyceride levels or both, as evident either prior to hospitalization or during it) and hypertension (systolic blood pressure greater than 150 mm/Hg or diastolic blood pressure greater than 90 mm/Hg or both, once more documented either during or prior to hospitalization) as additional risk factors influencing longer-term survival.

Data on long-term outcome extending over nine years following survived myocardial infarction were reported by Martin et al. (1983). The base sample for this study consisted of a consecutive series of patients between 30 and 69 years of age with confirmed diagnoses of myocardial infarction admitted to all coronary-care units in a single city over a one-year sampling period. The sample gave close to a complete representation of myocardial infarction within the sampling frame and provided a cohort for the prospective examination of 666 patients who had survived the first 28 days following myocardial infarction. Of these, 88% were alive at one year after the onset of illness, 67% at five years, and 52% at the final nine-year follow-up.

Of the 54 variables initially chosen for examination, 19 were considered to be of sufficient demographic, biological, or cardiological interest to warrant inclusion in both univariate and multivariate predictive statistics. Univariate analysis revealed 10 variables that were statistically associated with long-term outcome after myocardial infarction. These included age (the older the patient the greater the relative risk of death); a past history of myocardial infarction, angina pectoris, or stroke prior to the presenting illness; the presence of diabetes and hypertension, also prior to the present illness; the presence of sinus tachycardia (heart rate greater than 104 beats per minute); cardiac failure on admission to coronary care; and the complications of cardiac failure and reversible arrhythmias in the first 28 days following myocardial infarction. Among these variables, the highest relative risks were attached to prior history of stroke and to patients in the older age groups (65 to 69 years).

Multivariate analyses of the data confirmed these results, though prior cardiovascular or cerebrovascular disease this time produced the greatest relative risk of death. In addition, the patients' gender emerged as a significant prognostic factor, with males having a relative risk of 1.37 compared with female patients.

These prospective studies would seem to indicate then that two broad categories of cardiological variables, the one relating to a history of cardiovascular or cerebrovascular disease prior to the onset of myocardial infarction, the other relating to cardiovascular complications typically involving arrhythmias and heart failure experienced during the early stages of recovery after myocardial infarction, contribute both singly and collectively toward explaining a substantial part of the variance in recurrent myocardial infarction, whether survived or not. A number of attempts have been made to develop the predictive potential of such variables in such a way as to allow the calculation of numerical indices of prognosis designed to reflect an individual patient's chances of recurrent myocardial infarction into the future. Two of the more prominent clinical instruments resulting from such exercises have been the Peel Index (Peel, Semple, Wang, Lancaster, & Dall, 1960) and the Norris Index (Norris et al., 1970). In the latter of these, nine variables representing the area of demographic characteristics, preinfarction risk, location of the present infarction, and complications experienced during hospitalization were examined in relation to the three-year mortality of 757 consecutive patients admitted to coronary care with a documented myocardial infarction. Three-year mortality accounted for 33% of the initial cohort.

Five factors, namely location of myocardial infarction, systolic blood pressure on admission, and preadmission presence of diabetes, obesity and hypertension were not found to be statistically related to three-year mortality, though location of the myocardial infarction was shown to be an important factor in predicting short-term survival. The factors of patient's age, heart size, condition of lung fields (reflecting pulmonary congestion and a history of previous myocardial infarction) did, however, predict long-term mortality to a significant degree. A discriminant analysis allowed numerical weightings to be attached to the importance of these factors, with pulmonary congestion (lung fields on x-ray) emerging as the most powerful predictor of long-term outcome. Three-year mortality for patients without pulmonary congestion was 23%. Where venous congestion was evident, the mortality rose to 32%, while 64% of patients with interstitial edema or pulmonary edema did not survive to three years.

The next most important factor was that of age, with younger age groups achieving appreciably higher survival rates than older age groups. Age has traditionally been regarded as an important prognostic feature following myocardial infarction. Patients under 50 years of age at onset of the illness show an annual mortality rate of approximately 5%, whereas patients over 50 typically die at twice this rate (Willerson et al., 1982).

A history of previous myocardial infarction followed in importance as a predictor of long-term survival, with patients having experienced a previous event being at significantly higher risk of death over three years than patients for whom the present event was the first documented myocardial infarction. Finally, heart size as assessed by a standard chest x-ray taken within 24 hours of admission to hospital was a significant predictor of three-year mortality, with those having a doubtfully or definitely enlarged heart showing a higher risk than those for whom the heart size was normal.

A numerical index designed to reflect the chances of long-term survival was obtained by multiplying the presence and extent of the risk variable by a weight derived from the discriminant function analysis representing the importance of that variable in predicting risk. Longitudinal examination of the predictive power of the resultant coronary prognostic index scoring less than four had a three-year mortality approximating only 3%, while 78% of those with an index of 12 or more on admission to hospital had died within three years. Data such as these allow the conclusion that prognostic indices reflect, in a general sense, the level of severity of myocardial infarction.

The value of prognostic indicators is twofold. Firstly, they allow the physician to obtain an overview of the chances of survival and, moreover, to pinpoint those areas of cardiological concern which might militate against long-term survival. With this in mind, appropriate interventions may be initiated at a medical level to remove the risk of extension of the myocardial infarction in the short term after the onset of the illness (Willerson et al., 1982) and so to improve chances of long-term survival following discharge from hospital. Secondly, however, the use of coronary prognostic indices is of considerable value in research studies evaluating the effectiveness of a whole range of interventions following myocardial infarction, whether these be medical or behavioral, because failure to adequately control for the physiological severity of the myocardial infarction may result in errors of interpretation of outcome data to do with subsequent coronary morbidity and mortality. While it is not suggested that each patient scheduled for psychological intervention be labeled with a coronary prognostic index, and while the mere existence of this index may have serious implications for those involved in the management of the patient at any level, the value of such information where intervention strategies are to be systematically evaluated cannot be disregarded.

Evidence of the kind cited in the preceding pages of this chapter indicates that the myocardium, once compromised by recent acute myocardial infarction, is both vulnerable to and may be the focus of life-threatening physiological dysfunctions in the early period after the onset of illness. To this extent, factors to do with the nature and location of the myocardial infarction and the physiological vulnerability of the myocardium will play an overriding role in determining the process of outcome at this stage of the illness. As will be apparent from previous chapters, the risk of death or protracted illness, either from disruptions to the ventricular rhythm or subsequent myocardial infarction, appear to be concentrated at this point. The compromised integrity of the myocardium may, of course, also operate to influence a whole range of outcomes well into the period of occupational and social rehabilitation. The time course of rehabilitation and reintegration into pre-morbid social and occupational patterns does, however, allow the emergence of a set of influences more diverse than those related to the degree of damage sustained by the myocardium and its circulation.

3.   THE PERSISTENCE OF PRE-MORBID RISK FACTORS

The role of the traditional physiological and metabolic risk factors of hypertension, high serum cholesterol (perhaps reflected in obesity) and cigarette smoking in predicting the initial occurrence of coronary heart disease has been consistently documented in major epidemiological studies (see Chapter 1). Moreover, a number of extensive community studies aimed at the control of coronary heart disease through the modification of these risk factors, notably the North Karelia study in Finland (World Health Organization, 1981), the multiple risk factor intervention trial in the U.S.A. (Multiple Risk Factor Intervention Trial Research Group, 1982), and the World Health Organization European collaborative trial in the multifactorial prevention of coronary heart disease (Kornitzer, De Backer, Dramaix, Kittel, Thilly, Graffar & Vuylsteek, 1983; Rose, Tunstall-Pedoe, & Heller, 1983) have provided guarded if variable support for the idea that the control of risk factors contributes to the primary prevention of coronary heart disease.

   The issue of secondary prevention by means of risk-factor control is rather more contentious. Evidence from large cohort prospective studies of secondary occurrence have implicated hypertension at presentation (Martin et al., 1983), obesity, and both elevated serum cholesterol and triglycerides at presentation (Marmor et al., 1982) and cigarette smoking (Wilhelmsen, Wilhelmsen, Vedin, & Elmfeldt, 1982) as consistent contributors to recurrent myocardial infarction among long-term survivors of an initial event. The World Health Organization European Collaborative Study on rehabilitation and comprehensive secondary prevention after heart attack (World Health Organization, 1973, 1983) has extended data such as these into a large sample study directed toward the control of physiological and metabolic risk factors, and the evaluation of these measures in the secondary prevention of coronary heart disease.

   This study involved a cohort of 3,184 survivors of a first myocardial infarction drawn from 24 participating centers across Europe and in Israel. On recruitment into the study all patients were randomly allocated to one of two groups. The first involved intensive intervention utilizing the highest possible level of available local services and aiming toward the control of high blood pressure, serum lipids, weight and cigarette smoking where indicated by the individual patient's needs. The other group involved only the provision of routine medical care; and while patients were not denied any form of available treatment, the intensity of intervention and the specific aims of risk-factor control were not evident to the degree to be seen in the intervention group. Thus, the two groups were distinguished both by the level of intervention (to control risk factors) and the systematic approach with which intervention was invoked. Patients were subjected, where possible, to routine follow-up medical examinations at 12, 24, and 36 months after the initial heart attack, with mortality data being sought for nonsurvivors. Follow-up rates over three years, including data on coronary mortality during the follow-up period, averaged 78%, though this varied widely from one study center to another.

Taking three-year coronary mortality as the end point, intensive intervention aimed at risk-factor control appears to have very little to offer, with only one of the 24 participating study centers reporting lower mortality in patients being given the intervention program. The evidence is a little more clear when coronary morbidity is used as the end point, with nine participating studies reporting higher levels of subsequent myocardial infarction for the control group than for those offered intensive intervention. Seven study centers, however, reported the reverse effect. There was wide variation between study centers in rates of return to work over the three year follow-up period and no center reported a significant benefit of risk-factor intervention on the number of patients returning to work over this period.

These results are clearly disappointing. A number of aspects of the study design including variable compliance rates, logistic difficulties of between-center collaboration, failure by some centers to adequately implement the intervention programs, and insufficient sample sizes and follow-up periods have been seen to contribute to the equivocal outcomes. The more fundamental difficulty, however, lies in the fact that following myocardial infarction, the cardiovascular system is both physiologically and anatomically compromised and the activity of factors seen to contribute to the progressive but protracted process of coronary artery disease is unlikely to override in importance, particularly in the short term, the influence of acute complications arising from the compromised integrity of the myocardium and the coronary circulation. Put another way, cardiological outcome, at least after myocardial infarction, may be more a function of the capacity of the cardiovascular system to cope with acute challenges than of the further slow progression of presumably pre-existing coronary-artery disease.

Clearly, this rather simple account does not do justice to the situation. A factor such as the level of serum cholesterol, which acts to influence coronary risk by way of facilitating atherosclerotic deposits in the coronary arteries over a protracted period, will be likely to exert a far less acute effect on the cardiovascular system than a factor such as cigarette smoking which increases risk of myocardial infarction through the combined effects of myocardial stimulation by nicotine and depletion of myocardial oxygen because of increased concentrations of carbon monoxide in the blood. The finding that traditional risk factors had little to do with the process of returning to work is not surprising. This end point occurs sufficiently late after myocardial infarction to allow the influence of such factors as social and emotional maladjustment to assume determining roles and, moreover, if the presence of risk factors is related to speed or success of returning to work, it is more likely to be linked to this outcome through recurrent cardiac disease or medical advice to retire than through the presence of physiological or metabolic irregularities per se.

4.   DEMOGRAPHIC CHARACTERISTICS

Evidence on the demographic correlates of outcome has been more incidental than primary. Both clinical and epidemiological studies have consistently documented age as a determinant of outcome (Willerson et al., 1982), particularly with regard to morbidity and mortality in the year or two following myocardial infarction, though it is as likely that age as an influence is mediated by some factor such as extent of coronary-artery disease as it is that it acts as an independent risk factor for recurrent heart attack. Sex, too, has emerged as an incidental correlate of recurrence in epidemiological studies. However, the evidence here is not consistent, with males at higher risk of long-term recurrence (Martin et al., 1983) but females apparently at higher risk of short-term recurrence (Marmor et al., Roberts, 1982). These findings must clearly be viewed within the context that females have a significantly lower overall risk of coronary heart disease than males (Johnson, 1977).

The influence of educational level on outcome has also been documented in a series of studies using large cohorts. Men with less than eight years' schooling were shown to have three times the rate of recurrent myocardial infarction of those with more than eight years' schooling (Weinblatt, Ruberman, Goldberg, Frank, Shapiro, & Chaudhary, 1978), and this finding could not be accounted for simply by a combination of other risk factors (Ruberman, Weinblatt, Goldberg, & Chaudhary, 1983). The effect was evident, however, only among men who were shown on electrocardiographic examination to suffer from premature ventricular beats, and the phenomenon appeared to be associated with the presence of psychosocial stress (Ruberman et al., 1983).

Associations between more composite indices of social class and outcome have also been documented, with patients of lower social class being most strongly represented among those with poor occupational outcomes (Croog & Levine, 1977) and also with higher levels of coronary morbidity and mortality following myocardial infarction (Kottke, Young, & McCall, 1980). However, as with studies involving education alone, the effect may well reflect co-morbidity, with lower-class patients being denied interventions available to higher-class patients, perhaps due to the imposition of financial barriers to medical care (Kottke et al., 1980), their poorer capacity to articulate concerns and symptoms, or to understand and comply with medical instructions.

Associations between demographic characteristics of survivors of myocardial infarction and both short- and long-term outcomes are, therefore, broadly evident in the literature. The evidence would suggest, however, that these effects are mediated through more direct indicators of cardiovascular efficiency. For example, the level of disease in coronary arteries or the presence of ventricular arrhythmias. Moreover, since it is these mediating factors rather than demographic variables themselves, which are open to potential modification, research efforts in the future might be directed to a closer identification of the factors linking the patients' demographic characteristics with outcome. This is perhaps more pertinent to recurrent coronary events as outcomes than to such indices of outcome as return to work (Croog & Levine, 1977).

5.   THE TYPE A BEHAVIOR PATTERN

Causal associations between the Type A Behavior Pattern and risk of first myocardial infarction are now consistently in evidence in the epidemiological literature and will be reported more fully in other chapters of this book. Those persons with the behavior pattern appear to have around twice the risk of coronary heart disease, all other risk factors being accounted for, of those for whom Type A behavior is absent. As Razin (1982) has so succinctly put it, there is "... ample reason to believe that the Type A Behavior Pattern does not stop at the door of the coronary care unit." One might, therefore expect the possession of Type A behavior to be as relevant a determinant of recurrent myocardial infarction as of the initial event. Somewhat surprisingly, then, few studies have addressed this issue.

In a prospective investigation of 3,000 participants in the Western Collaborative Group Study it was found that scores on a self-reported scale of the Type A Behavior Pattern distinguished between men with single and men with recurrent myocardial infarctions, with scores for those with recurrent illness being significantly higher than those recorded by their single infarction counterparts (Jenkins et al., 1971). These results were confirmed in a later examination of the same cohort of subjects (Jenkins et al., 1976). In this report, the Type A Behavior Pattern was shown to be an independent predictor of recurrent myocardial infarction unrelated to the presence of serum cholesterol, cigarette smoking, or blood pressure. The strength of association between Type A behavior and recurrent myocardial infarction was, in fact, stronger than that for either serum-cholesterol levels or cigarette smoking.

These data build on similar results reported by Rosenman, Friedman, and Jenkins (1967) and have encouraged the development of a "recurrence scale" (Jenkins, 1978) in which items from one self-report scale of the Type A Behavior Pattern (the Jenkins Activity Survey) are being examined in an attempt to predict risk of recurrent infarction among those who have survived an initial event. Such data have also encouraged the initiation of large-scale attempts to modify Type A behavior following myocardial infarction, in an attempt to reduce the risk of secondary occurrence (Powell, Friedman, Thoresen, Gill, & Ulmer, 1984) though this work will be discussed in a later chapter.

Not all studies of the role of Type A behavior in recurrent myocardial infarction have, however, been equally positive. Case, Heller, and Shamai (1983) failed to find any association between the two. The major evidence, albeit from the one cohort of subjects (the Western Collaborative Group Study) does, however, support a causal role for this behavior pattern in predicting secondary heart attack.

6.   PSYCHOLOGICAL DISTRESS

Psychological distress associated with the experience of myocardial infarction is widespread (Byrne, 1979). The nature and course of emotional responses to myocardial infarction have been discussed in a previous chapter and need not be further expanded here. The anxiety and depression reported by patients recovering from myocardial infarction can, however, be expected to influence outcome on two general levels. Firstly, as Lown et al. (1980) have pointed out, a considerable body of evidence indicates that the higher nervous system modifies the electrical activity of the heart and the neurophysiological correlates of intense emotion may act to trigger ventricular arrhythmias resulting in reinfarction or sudden death. The liberation of catecholamines into the myocardium during times of emotional distress (Frankenhaeuser, 1979) might also be seen as a pathway of influence between emotions and cardiovascular functioning. Both these factors can be seen as potential determinants of cardiological outcome, and because the evidence on the time course of severe emotional distress places this in the first few days or weeks after myocardial infarction, its effects are most likely to be seen sooner rather than later in the course of recovery when the myocardium is vulnerable to insult from challenges of a physiological or chemical nature.

Secondly, emotional distress, if it is prolonged, may also act to influence occupational rehabilitation, either by generating uncertainty regarding the ability of the cardiovascular system to withstand the demands of the occupational situation (Byrne, 1979) or, if the emotional state be predominantly one of depression, by producing a situation of demoralization, hopelessness, and low motivation (Cay et al., 1976). The influence of psychological distress on occupational outcome is most likely to be seen later rather than sooner in the course of recovery, because successful return to work as an index of outcome does not typically occur for some weeks or months following the onset of illness.

Evidence relating psychological distress to outcome following myocardial infarction can be drawn from a number of studies. Ruberman et al. (1984) undertook a prospective investigation of 2,320 male survivors of acute myocardial infarction for whom extensive psychosocial data were available at the time of initial hospitalization. These patients also underwent a controlled 24-hour period of electrocardiographic monitoring during which susceptibility toward premature ventricular beats was noted. Follow-up examination of these men revealed that those classified as being socially isolated within peer groups and experiencing unduly high levels of life stress after illness had more than four times the risk of sudden cardiac death in the period immediately after myocardial infarction as those with low levels of stress and appropriate social integration. As had been previously reported, high levels of stress and social isolation were most prevalent among the least-educated men (Ruberman et al., 1983). This risk was independent of the presence of premature ventricular beats reported during the initial hospitalization, though earlier evidence (Lown et al., 1980), would certainly support the involvement of ventricular arrhythmias in the mediation between psychological distress and cardiac morbidity and mortality after initial heart attack.

A multivariate study of predictors of outcome in a smaller cohort of Scottish patients (Philip et al., 1979; Philip et al., 1981) ventured more widely in its consideration of outcomes than the simple index of recurrent coronary morbidity or mortality. These authors saw outcomes as encompassing (a) cardiological complications and recurrent myocardial infarction as measured by medical examination, (b) occupational and social rehabilitation and the emergence of psychological symptoms as measured by a psychiatric assessment, and (c) perceptions of encountered difficulties in the home and work environments as measured by patients' self-reported experiences.

Predictor variables in this study consisted of measures of psychological distress obtained during the first few days of hospitalization; these were related, by means of a multivariate predictive equation, to outcome variables assessed one year after the initial hospitalization in a cohort of 72 patients. Psychological distress evident soon after myocardial infarction significantly predicted a range of outcomes; however these had predominantly to do with the persistence of psychological distress into the year following myocardial infarction and the emergence of self-perceived difficulties related to incomplete rehabilitation and adjustment. Outcome, as measured by cardiovascular complication, reinfarction, or failure to return to work was not successfully predicted by psychological state immediately following heart attack. Similar results have been found in other studies (Mayou, 1984); though by contrast both Mulcahy (1976) and Diederiks, van der Sluijs, Weeda, and Schobre (1983) found failure to return to work to be more strongly related to psychological distress following myocardial infarction than to the extent of the infarction itself (as measured by a prognostic index).

A broadly based, prospective examination of the psychological determinants of outcome conceptualized within the framework of illness behavior was reported by Byrne et al. (1981). The independent variables in this study consisted of eight descriptive factors representing a broad range of cognitive, behavioral, and emotional responses to myocardial infarction. These factors have been described in some detail in a previous chapter (see also Byrne & Whyte, 1978). Outcome variables represented the three categories of (a) recurrent coronary morbidity or subsequent mortality, (b) success and speed of return to work, and (c) patient reports of self-perceived well-being and satisfaction with progress following discharge from hospital. In this respect, the outcome variables were not dissimilar from those used by Philip et al. (1981). The cohort for the study consisted of 120 survivors of a first documented myocardial infarction with data on illness behavior being collected within two weeks of first hospitalization and measures of outcome taken both eight months and 24 months after leaving hospital.

No aspect of illness behavior evident within the two-week period following myocardial infarction distinguished those patients who would enjoy a cardiologically uneventful eight-month outcome from those who would at some time during the intervening period experience a further myocardial infarction warranting readmission to a coronary-care unit and survive this recurrent event. However, when patients with a subsequent myocardial infarction resulting in death were added to the outcome group, two aspects of previously manifested illness behavior were associated with this composite index of subsequent morbidity and mortality. Patients with recurrent coronary events, whether survived or not, were more likely to be characterized by a recognition of the presence of serious life stress in the period preceding the initial myocardial infarction and of attributing the first illness to this stress. Moreover, these patients were more likely than others to have expressed, soon after the first myocardial infarction, an attitude of enhanced concern for aspects of bodily function and well-being.

Associations between the experience of life stress and the occurrence of myocardial infarction have, of course, been documented in the past (Byrne & Whyte, 1980), raising the possibility that patients characterized by this aspect of illness behavior may have been among that group with an accumulation of stressful life events occurring prior to the original myocardial infarction. It begs the speculation, moreover, that for these individuals, stressful life events continued into the period of recovery and rehabilitation and contributed to the subsequent coronary event by the same mechanisms linking life events with the initial illness. Concurrent measures of the experience of stressful life events during the follow-up period confirmed this suggestion by showing that patients with recurrent coronary events, either survived or otherwise, did indeed accumulate a significantly higher number of self-reported distressing life events in the follow-up period than did those who enjoyed a recovery free from the intrusion of distressing life experience. These findings are much in accord with the work of Ruberman et al. (1984) relating life stress following myocardial infarction to a recurrence of the event.

The small but noticeable increase in risk of recurrent heart attack associated with feelings of somatic concern soon after the original myocardial infarction is not surprising. While it may reflect little more than that those patients experiencing anxiety centering on the integrity of cardiovascular functioning may have also been those patients who sustained the most severe myocardial infarction (and who are therefore at greatest risk of recurrence), the documented physiological influence of anxiety on cardiovascular function (Lown et al., 1980) would seem to provide a plausible mediating pathway between perceptions of emotional distress, whatever the thematic content, and risk of subsequent coronary events.

The findings of Byrne et al. (1981) were strengthened even further when frequency of medical consultations was used as an outcome variable. While this can not, strictly speaking, be considered a measure of cardiological outcome since such medical consultations did not necessarily reflect recurrent events, it may indicate that somatic anxiety surrounding the initial myocardial infarction sensitizes patients to the presence and perceptions of minor cardiovascular symptoms in the later stages of their recovery.

Aspects of illness behavior evident soon after myocardial infarction also predicted return to work in the eight month follow-up period. Anxiety was prominent in this respect, though the variable of interest rested more with generalized anxiety than with focused concern regarding physiological functioning. More prominently, however, it was found that those failing to return to work in the eight month follow-up period had, soon after the original myocardial infarction, shown a greater readiness to accept the sick role (Parsons, 1951) than those who would subsequently return to gainful employment. Once more, the most obvious explanation for this finding is that patients readily adopting sick-role behaviors are those who are most severely ill—and, therefore, those who are least likely to be able to return to work. Patients rarely, however, have access to evidence that allows them to make such objective and accurate estimates of the severity of their own pathology. Rather, they tend to make subjective and frequently distorted judgments of their condition based on perceptions of sensations emanating from the location of the pathology, attitudes to illness, individual personality traits, and the like. Insofar as myocardial infarction is concerned, the evidence suggests that psychological responses to illness are, by and large, not strongly influenced by the objective severity of the infarction (Vetter et al., 1977).

This apparent association between the extent of coronary pathology and measures of outcome is most particularly to be seen with regard to return to work. The most consistent finding seems to be that failure to achieve adequate occupational rehabilitation is due more to adverse psychological responses to illness than it is to the objective severity of the myocardial infarction (Cay et al., 1973; Mulcahy, 1976). A finer examination of patterns of return to work revealed no association between any aspect of illness behavior and the need to change the nature of work among those who returned to active employment. Nor was there any association between return to work and the nature of the job, whether it was sedentary, light physical, or moderate to heavy physical.

Illness behavior soon after myocardial infarction also appeared to influence some aspects of psychosocial outcome and reports of subjectively perceived satisfaction with progress and well-being eight months after the event. Patients reporting a deterioration in the pattern of their social lives during the eight month follow-up period had expressed, soon after myocardial infarction, a greater level of concern with the integrity of cardiovascular function than had patients who saw their social lives as being unaffected by the myocardial infarction. The same patients were also characterized by significantly higher levels of generalized affective disturbance than were patients whose social lives had remained unaltered (Byrne, 1982a). Measures of psychosocial outcome have frequently been neglected in prospective studies of prognosis following myocardial infarction either because of supposed problems of measurement or because studies with specifically medical objectives have viewed psychosocial outcome in its various forms as too trivial a set of events to be concerned with. This omission has been seen as regrettable (Mayou et al., 1978) in view of the surprisingly high numbers of patients who, although they experienced cardiologically uneventful outcomes, nonetheless reported crippling levels of emotional stress and severe social incapacity well into the period of recovery and rehabilitation (Mayou, 1984). Such social incapacity, which not uncommonly generalizes to difficulties in occupational rehabilitation, has been seen to stem from a failure of emotional adjustment at the time of the original myocardial infarction (Mayou, 1984), and an unreasonable and unwarranted fear that damage sustained by the cardiovascular system at the time of the myocardial infarction will continue indefinitely to preclude any but the most incidental social encounters or lightest of occupational activities (Finlayson & McEwen, 1977; Byrne, 1982a). The persistence of such attitudes is curious when they may have been resolved soon after illness onset by the simple provision of information centering on the individual patient's fears and concerns regarding the causes and consequences of myocardial infarction.

A follow-up of this cohort of patients 24 months after the original myocardial infarction indicated that any influence of illness behavior which might have been evident on the various aspects of outcome at eight months had all but disappeared at two years (Byrne, 1982b). Such long-term investigations of the psychological determinants of outcome after myocardial infarction are not often undertaken but should be considered in view of the contention (Finlayson & McEwen, 1977) that the process of outcome continues to unfold well past one year after the onset of illness. The little evidence that is available would suggest, however, that if psychological responses to myocardial infarction are to have bearing on outcomes, the course of this influence will be evident sooner rather than later in the process of recovery and rehabilitation. The implications of this for intervention to alleviate potentially harmful psychological responses to myocardial infarction should be initiated as close as possible to the illness event rather than months away from it (Mayou, 1984).

The sources of psychological distress following myocardial infarction can be sought in a variety of areas. Myocardial infarction is a life-threatening illness, the outcome of which is frequently uncertain, at least in the eyes of the patient (Byrne et al., 1981). The dangers of recurrence and death or of protracted disability, whether actual or perceived (Doehrman, 1977), occupy a substantial amount of the patient's conscious thought. In the days soon after myocardial infarction, the patient is subject to intense medical scrutiny, frequently with the assistance of unfamiliar and personally intrusive medical technology, while confined within the completely foreign environment of the coronary-care unit. For some, at least, this experience reinforces feelings of uncertainty regarding the continuation of life and health and may trigger the onset of acute emotional distress (Dominian & Dobson, 1969), while for others the experience of a coronary-care-unit admission may act to reassure the patient of the availability of care (Razin, 1982); the coronary-care unit as a psychological hazard should not be underestimated (Hackett, Cassem, & Wishnie, 1968).

Even among those who are comforted by the medical scrutiny afforded to them in the coronary-care unit, transfer from this facility to a general medical ward has been found to be associated with both increases in levels of emotional distress and with potential medical complications to recovery (Hackett et al., 1968) unless the patient has been adequately prepared by way of the provision of information regarding the transfer and the reasons for it (Klein, Kliner, Zipes, Troyer, & Wallace, 1968). Interestingly, the same effect does not appear to result from early discharge from hospital, at least among those with uncomplicated myocardial infarction (Ahlmark, Ahlberg, Saetre, Haglund, & Korsgren, 1979), though psychological preparation for discharge from hospital is more commonly undertaken than that for discharge from intensive coronary care. With this contrast in mind, it might be of interest to compare levels of affective distress in patients with complicated myocardial infarction, and the possible effect this might have on response to hospital discharge and on outcome.

Of course, neither survival nor the continued integrity of the cardiovascular system represent the only sources of anxiety for the survivor of myocardial infarction. Uncertainties surrounding the re-establishment of social roles and relationships (Mayou et al., 1978), a return to active employment (Finlayson & McEwen, 1977), the need to face interpersonal and family conflicts existing prior to myocardial infarction (Croog & Levine, 1977), and perceived difficulties associated with the resumption of active sex life (Wagner, 1974) have all been cited as sources of potential distress in patients recovering from myocardial infarction. While the effective use of denial has been found to circumvent undue emotional distress at least among some patients (Croog et al., 1971; Gentry, Foster, & Haney, 1972) and while the mobilization of social support appears to offer some protection in the fact of emotional distress among some patients (Razin, 1982), the fact remains that sizable numbers of patients surviving myocardial infarction experience emotional distress of a moderate to severe degree, and this emotional distress may work to influence outcome, whether at the cardiological, occupational, or social levels.

7.   OVERVIEW

The diversity of evidence bearing on the determination of outcome following myocardial infarction does not reduce either to a simple or unified model of this process. The size and location of the myocardial infarction itself, together with the presence of cardiological complications in the period shortly after, are clearly of crucial importance in predicting outcome, particularly insofar as this is defined by subsequent coronary morbidity and mortality in the short term, though to the extent that the capacity and efficiency of cardiovascular system is irreversibly compromised to a greater or lesser degree by heart attack, these factors are also likely to have an influence on occupational readjustment in the longer term. The evidence, particularly from long-term studies of outcome is, however, equally persuasive that immediate psychological responses to myocardial infarction, and perhaps their prolongation, can also bear on oucome. While such factors are rather more difficult to conceptualize and to define than others do with the pathophysiology of the cardiovascular system, prospective evidence nonetheless supports the causal influence of emotional and behavioral responses to myocardial infarction on each of the diverse outcomes of that clinical event. While mechanisms for such a course of influence remain unclear, both experimental and clinical evidence indicates the essential involvement of the central nervous system (Lown et al., 1980) in the mediation of this process.

CHAPTER 5

Psychological Intervention Following Myocardial Infarction

1. THE ACUTE MANAGEMENT OF THE CARDIAC PATIENT

The diagnosis of myocardial infarction, or indeed a firm clinical suspicion of that state, initiates a series of medical actions designed, in the first instance, to sustain life and, in the longer term, to promote recovery and rehabilitation. In the acute stage of illness, lasting between three and seven days, the former of these is emphasized and the activities are centered on the coronary-care unit. Patients with unequivocal or suspected myocardial infarction are therefore immediately on admission to the coronary-care unit placed under continuous monitoring to detect potentially fatal irregularities in the electrical functioning of the myocardium and ceaseless visual observation by nursing staff to detect immediately the presence of signs and symptoms indicating physical distress. Such functions as heart rate and blood pressure are frequently checked, sometimes using automated equipment, and regular examinations of blood chemistry are routine. This intensive medical attention is designed to provide coronary-care staff with the most immediate information possible on the patient's physical condition so that irregularites, when detected, may be corrected without delay.

It was suggested in the previous chapter that such concentrated medical scrutiny, together with a physical environment abounding in the products of medical and technological achievement produce, for at least some vulnerable patients, the ideal conditions for the development of emotional distress (Hackett et al., 1968). There has also been some question in the past (Mather et al., 1971) as to whether management in the coronary-care unit offers appreciable long-term advantages to the patient with myocardial infarction relative to those managed in the home, though the issue is highly contentious (Rose, 1975). Two recent and very extensive reviews of the available literature (Doehrman, 1977; Razin, 1982) strongly favor the conclusion that there is no consistent support for the proposition that admission to a coronary-care unit, attachment to an electrocardiograph monitoring device, or the observation of medical procedures concerned with the intensive care of other cardiac patients produce either short- or long-term emotional distress in the large majority of patients with mycardial infarction. There is little doubt now, however, that the provision of intensive coronary care produced marked and measurable decreases in postmyocardial infarction mortality rates (Crampton, Aldridge, Gascho, Miles, & Stillerman, 1975; Pole et al., 1977). On balance, then, the value of intensive coronary care following myocardial infarction would appear to be unchallenged. A comprehensive account of the medical management of patients in the acute phase of myocardial infarction has been written by Flaherty and Weisfeldt (1977). Neither this account nor any comparable one, however, devotes suitable time and attention to the care of the patient's emotional needs during this phase of illness.

The medical management of the patient with myocardial infarction, while at a somewhat less intensive level, is continued into the recovery phase following discharge from the coronary-care unit to a general medical ward. It is usually only after discharge from hospital, however, that management on a broader scale is initiated to allow the patient to proceed as rapidly as possible through to an unhindered social and occupational life. In some instances, this management consists of no more than a regular series of physical examinations conducted by the cardiologists to assess the state of the patient's cardiovascular system. In other instances, it involves the use of a structured rehabilitation program designed to encompass the whole range of needs which the patient will have on leaving hospital.

The World Health Organization (1981) defined rehabilitation to include all measures aimed at reducing the impact of disabling and handicapping conditions and at enabling the disabled and handicapped to achieve social integration. In a review of rehabilitation programs presently available for survivors of myocardial infarction, Kallio (1982) included in that definition the aim of preventing further coronary heart disease and went on to add that while the social and occupational rehabilitation of the patient will usually be achieved within a year after myocardial infarction and often after a relatively short program of active rehabilitation, the secondary preventive measures may have to be continued much longer.

One major focus for medical rehabilitation has been the provision of exercise programs leading to submaximal physical exertion. The primary focus of interest underlying this seems to be the influence which graded aerobic exercise might have on the development of collateral blood vessels within the myocardium and, therefore, on the maximization of cardiac efficiency. Stern and Cleary (1981) undertook a study of 784 men under the age of 64 who had suffered a first myocardial infarction. These men were admitted to a six-week, low-level exercise program where exercise intensity was limited to a maximum of 72% of age-predicted heart rate. They found that low-level exercise was sufficient to stimulate positive though largely unspecified psychosocial and vocational changes among some subjects; however this was limited to an upper-middle-class volunteer population. In a later report which considered only the 651 men who completed the exercise program (Stern & Cleary, 1982), it was found that, with minimal exceptions, there were no differences between exercise and control groups in terms of the degree of psychosocial benefit in measures at a number of follow-up periods ranging up to two years after myocardial infarction. In a similar study undertaken by Mayou, MacMahon, Sleight, and Florencio (1981) it was found that structured exercise following myocardial infarction afforded no particular advantages in terms of psychological outcome, physical activity, or satisfaction with leisure or work up to 12 weeks after the heart attack. At this point, patients in the exercise group were reported to be more enthusiastic about their treatment and to have achieved higher work levels on exercise testing than those in the control group. However, at 18-month follow-up there appeared to be no benefits at all to be seen for patients given earlier exercise training and Mayou and his colleagues were led to conclude that while exercise training increased confidence during the early stages of convalescence, the overall results showed that rehabilitation of this kind is of little benefit to cardiac function, everyday-life activities, or the patient's emotional state. Kallio (1982) arrived at similar conclusions following a review of early activation and physical exercise programs after myocardial infarction and pointed out, in particular, that exercise rehabilitation evaluated by controlled studies has shown no particular advantages in terms of increased life expectancy after myocardial infarction. Thus, while the rationale of physical exercise after myocardial infarction is physiologically sound, and while exercise programs still appear to be included in more broadly based rehabilitation packages, the evidence to date would not support physical exercise as a crucial focus for attention in intervention after myocardial infarction. This view has been placed on record by a report on cardiac rehabilitation from the Royal College of Physicians (London, 1975), where it was concluded that structured exercise training after myocardial infarction did not appear to produce notable advantages in terms of long-term survival.

Many reports have appeared in the literature in the past decade documenting broadly based multifaceted programs of rehabilitation following myocardial infarction. These have involved a composite of strategies, and while physical exercise retraining has been prominent, the inclusion of elements of education about myocardial infarction and its consequences, general counseling of patients about the problems they might encounter following hospitalization, and the involvement of spouses in the counseling and education programs have added much to the scope of rehabilitation efforts. The majority of studies have been proscriptive and exhortative in nature, in the sense that while they have described the operation of rehabilitative programs, they have provided very little empirical data on which to base an assessment of the advantages to be gained from these programs. Only recently have these data been collected, perhaps in part response to the World Health Organization initiatives in the area of cardiac rehabilitation (World Health Organization, 1973), though studies designed to adequately evaluate the effectiveness of multifaceted programs of cardiac rehabilitation are complex, lengthy, and expensive.

Kallio et al. (1979) developed such a multifaceted intervention program focusing on education, exercise, and counseling and examined the benefits which its provision might bring to long-term (three year) morbidity, mortality, and return to work in a group of patients 65 years and younger who had suffered a first documented myocardial infarction. One-half of the 375 patients in the trial were randomly assigned to an intervention group involving systematic attention to each of the three areas of concern, while the other half were assigned to a control group and received routine medical care and follow-up only. The two groups were matched for age and for the distribution of various prognostic variables. Active rehabilitation commenced around four weeks after the myocardial infarction and involved a series of regular sessions extending over a period of approximately a year. At three-year follow-up, the cumulative coronary mortality was significantly lower in the intervention group (18.6%) than in the control group (29.4%), and this was due largely to a reduction of sudden deaths in the intervention group. The influence of rehabilitation seemed, therefore, to be most prominent during the first six months after myocardial infarction, underscoring the value of early rehabilitation efforts in the secondary prevention of coronary disease.

Salonen and Puska (1980) reported the results of a study involving 1,308 survivors of myocardial infarction aged 65 or less, of which 515 were assigned on a voluntary basis to a posthospital rehabilitation program. The rehabilitation activities were organized at the community outpatient level, the main components of the program being health education and submaximal exercise along with treatment aimed at the reduction of the known secondary risk factors. Invervention was undertaken in small groups at outpatient clinics and decentralized local group rehabilitation centers. Patient interest in rehabilitation and compliance with the directions of rehabilitation program were found to be high over the course of five-year follow-up. Moreover, in that period of time, patients in active rehabilitation programs sustained significantly fewer subsequent episodes of myocardial infarction and were less likely to apply for invalidity pensions than those who chose not to participate.

Takeuchi (1983) examined the effects of a rehabilitation program during hospitalization on the prognosis of 496 patients surviving myocardial infarction. Once more, the rehabilitation program involved education, exercise, and counseling; however, it commenced early during the patient's hospital stay and was short, intensive, and completed before the patient left the hospital. No outpaitent involvement was undertaken. A follow-up investigation after a period somewhat in excess of five years indicated a death rate from subsequent myocardial infarction of 8.4% in the intervention group and 27% in the control group. Rates of return to work were similarly distinct for the two groups, with 50.2% of rehabilitated patients resuming active employment over the follow-up period compared with 25% of patients in the nonrehabilitation control group.

Data such as these do, therefore, support the assertion by the International Society and Federation for Cardiology (1980) that planned and sustained intervention following myocardial infarction can substantially improve prognosis.

Following a critical evaluation of the literature, Kallio (1982) concluded the effects of an organized, relatively simple program of rehabilitation during the first three months after myocardial infarction produced significant benefits in terms of short-term survival and morbidity relative to patients for whom routine medical care was the only follow-up available. The evidence appeared to support the value of rapid and early intervention activity and suggested that outpatient rehabilitation, organized simply at a community level, was as effective a facilitator of outcome benefits as more sophisticated programs requiring inpatient care.

2. THE RATIONALE FOR PSYCHOLOGICAL INTERVENTION

There is now no serious doubt that psychological factors contribute, through a variety of paths, to the development of coronary-artery disease and the onset of myocardial infarction. It will also be clear from previous chapters, and particularly from Chapter 4, that a range of behavioral and psychological considerations bear on the processes of recovery and rehabilitation after myocardial infarction. This would seem to be true no matter what measure of outcome is considered. So, for example, it can be shown that the possession of Type A behavior is as strong a predictor of secondary myocardial infarction as it is of the primary illness event (Jenkins et al, 1976). Moreover, it would appear that at least some aspects of illness behavior following myocardial infarction may assume a maladaptive function and predispose to unsatisfactory outcomes (Byrne et al, 1981; Byrne, 1982). Indeed, it has been said that unsatisfactory patterns of emotional and behavioral adjustment to myocardial infarction can, under some circumstances, be more consistent determinants of outcome than the physical severity of the myocardial infarction itself (Mulcahy, 1976; Mayou et al., 1978b).

The widespread occurrence of distressing and sometimes disproportionately intense emotional responses to myocardial infarction is described in an earlier chapter. Evidence has also been presented to document associations between psychological factors and outcome, and a range of mechanisms through which this influence might become manifest have been suggested. In view of this demonstrated set of influences, the issue of the potential role for psychosocial and behavioral intervention following myocardial infarction becomes self-evident. Put more specifically, one is led to ask the question: Given the clear influence of psychological and behavioral factors on outcomes after myocardial infarction, might it be the case that intervention strategies appropriately designed to modify those aspects of emotion or behavior that have been shown to predispose to unsatisfactory outcomes could, for some individuals, lead both in the short term and long term to reductions in subsequent coronary morbidity and mortality and facilitate a more rapid readjustment to personal, social, and occupational environments?

These issues have not, by and large, been addressed by studies emphasizing the traditional models of cardiac rehabilitation. While there is a little evidence that such procedures as exercise and health education can have a beneficial effect on the individual's feelings of well-being and psychosocial adjustment following myocardial infarction (Stern & Cleary, 1981), empirical studies reporting a systematic evaluation of the effectiveness of psychological and behavioral intervention on the range of medical, occupation, and social outcomes after myocardial infarction have been sparse by comparison with studies evaluating the effectiveness of medical management and risk-factor reduction.

3. PSYCHOLOGICAL AND BEHAVIORAL MANAGEMENT AFTER MYOCARDIAL INFARCTION

3.1   The Acute Phase

The literature pertinent to psychological intervention in the acute phase following myocardial infarction can be divided roughly into two categories, the first involving exhortatory studies based on case report and clinical anecdote; the second presenting systematic interventions supported by evaluative empirical data. Doehrman (1977) reviewed 36 studies in the former of the two categories, of which 24 were concerned with intervention in the acute phase. This focused on the psychological management of the cardiac patient either in the intensive-coronary-care unit or in a general medical war prior to discharge from hospital. These reports (for they cannot be accorded the status of empirical studies) arose predominantly from medically qualified persons, though around 40% were written by professionals with qualifications in nursing, psychology, or occupational therapy. The range of interventions was broad and extended from simple education regarding recovery from coronary heart disease to counseling in order to alleviate the emotional distress surrounding myocardial infarction. While none of these papers presents anything that could pass for empirical evaluation, the consensus arising from them would appear to be that the many and varied interventions proposed by this professionally diverse range of authors all acted to the advantage of the patient, both in terms of occupational and psychosocial readjustment and (somewhat more tenuously) in terms of a reduction in subsequent coronary risk.

Following a similar review of the exhortatory and prescriptive literature, Razin (1982) set down a series of guidelines emerging from clinical experience aimed at maximizing the benefits of acute-phase psychological intervention. These guidelines were: (a) intervention should be detailed, repetitive, and educational in nature; (b) those intervening should take an open, honest approach to patients, showing both compassion and confidence in their own competence; (c) clinicians should be aware of the time course and specificity of patients' reactions to myocardial infarction; (d) anxiety and emotional stress should be treated supportively and thus minimized wherever possible; and (e) early physical mobilization should be encouraged. The organization of intervention along these lines should, as evidence quoted by Razin (1982) indicates, produce clinical and psychological benefits in the overall management of the survivor of myocardial infarction. While this prescriptive information is of some interest, a more substantive consideration of these reports will not be made here because, as Razin (1982) has said, "these guidelines emerge from clinical experiences and virtually none of them enjoys rigorously derived empirical supporting data." The value of this material—and the guidelines emerging from it—is, however, that it provides the clinical and procedural underpinnings for the more systematic and empirically evaluated studies to be now considered.

A small number of papers, though still based on uncontrolled case description and observation, have attempted to present somewhat more systematically collected information on psychological intervention following myocardial infarction. These papers have typically addressed specific problems arising during recovery and convalescent phases after hospitalization and have taken a predominantly psychoanalytic approach with emphasis on the exploration of both feelings and concerns. Bilodeau and Hackett (1971) discussed these within the broad groupings of fears about death from recurrent heart attack, loss of self-esteem resulting from diminished physical integrity and sexual activity, perhaps resulting from a fear of excessive physical exertion during intercourse. Group therapy (weekly over a period of 12 weeks) was undertaken with a small group of five patients and was aimed at the broad resolution of these difficulties. All patients remained free of distressing cardiac symptoms during the course of therapy and there was no recurrence of myocardial infarction in this 12-week period. Moreover, there was anecdotal evidence of the development among patients of a more adaptive psychological state during treatment. However, data were by way of anecdotal case report only and there was neither a control group nor a follow-up. A similar study by Mone (1970), in which 14 patients were offered weekly sessions of group psychotherapy spread over 10 weeks and designed to resolve emotional and family difficulties following the experience of myocardial infarction, reported systematic and sequential changes in the patients' psychological state as measured by several scales of the Minnesota Multiphasic Personality Inventory. However, once more, there was no control group or follow-up and, therefore, no data on the effectiveness of intervention on either recurrent myocardial infarction or occupational rehabilitation.

More intensive psychoanalytic treatment undertaken and evaluated by both Karstens and colleagues (Karstens, Kohle, & Ohlmeier, 1970; Ohlmeier, Karstens, & Kohle, 1973), and Hahn and Leisner (1970) aimed both at the emotional distress surrounding myocardial infarction and the intrapsychic conflict associated with the experience of the illness have reported beneficial effects of the intervention on measures of emotional and social outcome. Once more, however, the data have been derived from case anecdote, and neither control groups nor follow-up have been employed. The value of these studies is, therefore, not so much in terms of their contributions to an understanding of the influence of psychological intervention on outcome after myocardial infarction as it is on the elucidation of difficulties, conflicts, and concerns both among patients and their families that might impede the processes of recovery and rehabilitation and which might, by their nature, be amenable to psychological intervention. These issues have been taken up in a series of recent and worthwhile reviews (Frank, Hiller, & Kornfeld, 1979; Hackett, 1978; Soloff, 1979), and these establish the ground for more systematically implemented and evaluated psychological interventions.

3.2   Systematic Acute Phase Interventions

While there is a large observational and clinical literature on psychological interventions directed at the resolution of intrapsychic, emotional, and social difficulties associated with myocardial infarction (see Section 3.1), there has been an apparent reluctance to commence systematic or structured interventions directed toward the long-term recovery and rehabilitation of cardiac patients while the patient remains within the coronary-care unit or the inpatient hospital environment. Perhaps this is due to the fact that the patient remains acutely and sometimes dangerously ill, and the initiation of any activity other than that aimed directly at the protection of the cardiovascular system is seen as superfluous and unwarranted. It may be due also to the fact that the already crowded coronary-care-unit environment is unable to tolerate the routine presence of yet another care giver. While these issues of the organization of medical services are clearly important and to be respected, the fact remains that the patient's emotional and psychological state during the acute phase of recovery can have both immediate and long-term influences on ultimate outcome. Lynch, Thomas, Mills, Malinow, and Katcher (1974) showed that a range of emotional and social circumstances such as adverse psychological responses to illness or family visits could precipitate potentially dangerous cardiac arrhythmias among at least some cardiac patients, leading Razin (1982) to comment on the "exquisite sensitivity of the compromised heart to psychosocial stimuli." The potential and short-term consequences of failure to initiate psychological intervention in the early stages of recovery are, therefore, clear. The long-term consequence of unrecognized or untreated emotional distress or psychological maladaptation in the period immediately surrounding myocardial infarction are sufficiently well documented (Byrne et al., 1981; Byrne, 1982) to require little further comment. The need for early psychological intervention following myocardial infarction would, therefore, appear to be self-evident.

Stein, Murdaugh, and MacLeod (1969) offered brief supportive psychotherapy to a small number of patients experiencing pronounced emotional reactions to myocardial infarction on the grounds that such emotional reactions might prove noxious to the patient's cardiac state. The focus of the investigation was on the experience of undue emotional stress during the acute phase of recovery from myocardial infarction. While the provision of psychotherapy was varied according to the needs of individual patients and the study was uncontrolled, the authors reported that patients experienced both cardiological and psychological benefits from intervention at this early stage in their illness. The interpretation of data such as these does, however, pose difficulties, since the unsystematic presentation of psychotherapy does not allow a differential evaluation of its active elements and the absence of control groups limits inferences to be drawn from the data. Moreover, failure to make therapy consistent across patients muddies interpretation even further and precludes any real replication. A much more extensive and well controlled investigation into the effects of psychological intervention following myocardial infarction was reported by Gruen (1975). Patients in this study comprised those who had experienced a first myocardial infarction and were in the age range of 40 to 69 years. Patients with conspicuous psychological disorder under treatment were excluded from investigation. Eligible patients were seen in the first few days of admission to a coronary-care unit and were randomly assigned either to an intervention or control group until 35 patients had accumulated in each. Comparisons of a number of demographic and medical variables at the conclusion of the study indicated that the samples were matched for age, sex, marital status, and social class. They were also matched for severity and location of myocardial infarction. Patients in the intervention group were contacted either on the first or second day in the coronary-care unit and, after agreement to participate in the study, this was followed by regular half-hour sessions on five or six days a week until release from hospital. Gruen avoided the use of the term "psychologist" in patient contact and instead identified himself as a member of "the Department of Patient Care Improvement."

Psychological intervention, while essentially open ended, attempted to systematically establish a series of 10 therapeutic components which Gruen considered to be important both for the resolution of emotional distress following myocardial infarction and in the facilitation of adaptive behavior during the rehabilitation phase, leading to reintegration into work and society. These therapeutic components can be summarized as follows:

a. the establishment of rapport with the patient along what appeared to be Rogerian lines;
b. reassurance as to the essential normality of the patient's fear and concern in resonse to myocardial infarction;
c. an exploration and reinforcement of coping mechanisms already developed for use in the face of crisis, though perhaps not immediately apparent to the patient;

d. a recognition and reflection of the patient's present feelings and developing judgments regarding the myocardial infarction (that is, accurate empathy);

e. recognition and challenge of negative impressions and cognitions regarding myocardial infarction; for example, convictions of the inevitability of death or protracted disability and fear of remaining a burden on significant others for prolonged periods of time; provision of opportunities for the patient to explore these in a rational and supportive environment;

f. recognition of patient's desires to assimilate only particular kinds of information and the restriction of topics for discussion to those that the patient is prepared to accept;

g. encouragement of the patient to be confident and independent in seeking medical advice and to seek it from primary rather than secondary sources;

h. feedback and reassurance to the patient of the therapist's confidence in the patient's ability to cope with the challenge of myocardial infarction;

i. encouragement of the patient to face and resolve conflicts as they appeared;

j. continual reinforcement of pre-existing coping behaviors and resources already available to deal with crisis.

Control and intervention subjects were compared both at discharge from hospital and after a short follow-up period on a range of measures of cardiological, social, and emotional outcomes. The results indicated that distinct and significant outcome benefits arising from intervention were to be gained in a number of respects. Patients in the intervention group spent significantly fewer days in hospital, significantly fewer days in intensive care, and significantly fewer days on cardiac-monitoring equipment that did patients in the control group. Moreover, there were significantly fewer patients in the intervention group who experienced congestive heart failure as compared with those in the control group. Patients receiving psychological intervention also appeared to experience gains in the emotional sphere and reported significantly less anxiety and depression than did their control colleagues. These emotional benefits were carried through to the follow-up period.

This study is important in at least three respects. Firstly, psychological intervention was initiated early rather than later in the course of the patient's recovery. Secondly, the study was well designed and conducted and represents a serious scientific attempt to evaluate the effectiveness of early psychological intervention on outcome following myocardial infarction. The presentation of empirical data underscores the scientific credibility of the study. Thirdly, the results are particularly encouraging and indicate quite strongly that a range of cardiological and emotional benefits are to be gained by early psychological intervention after myocardial infarction.

Drawing on Gruen's important and pioneering work, Oldenburg and Perkins (1984) examined the influence of brief hospital-based psychological intervention among survivors of first myocardial infarction, beginning within a day or two of admission to coronary care and extending over the following seven to 10 days. Intervention was based on two assumptions, the first being that it should be offered early in the acute phase; the second being that it should serve the functions of support, education, and life-style change.

Patients admitted to a coronary-care unit with a first myocardial infarction were randomly assigned to one of three groups, which may be described as follows:

Group 1: These patients received daily sessions involving counseling, education about myocardial infarction and its risks and consequences, and training in systematic relaxation. Counseling, which was primarily supportive, served to allow the patient the opportunity of dealing with life-adjustment problems by reflection through the therapist using a client-centered approach and emphasizing the attainment of appropriate solutions to problems. Things that were specifically dealt with included fear of death, fear of developing chronic invalidity, anxiety about coping after hospitalization, anxiety about future sexual functioning, and pervasive depression. Education was designed to acquaint the patient with the basic causes of coronary heart disease and with the range of possible consequences following discharge from hospital. A passive, imaginal relaxation exercise was also taught in order not to overstress the vulnerable myocardium by the imposition of potentially dangerous isometric exercises (Davidson, Winchester, Taylor, Alderman, & Ingels, 1979).

Group 2: These patients received only the education and relaxation components given to patients in the first group, with no counseling being provided. Additional concentration on regular and routine relaxation exercises on a daily basis allowed the accumulation by this group of an equivalent intervention time to patients in Group 1.

Group 3: These patients formed a control group and received no treatment other than routine medical and nursing care.

All patients were seen individually and the education and relaxation material used in groups 1 and 2 was reinforced by the use of prerecorded audio cassette tapes. Patients were encouraged to retain these tapes following discharge from hospital, to continue relaxation exercises, and to involve their families both in relaxation and education.

A range of outcomes was assessed at the point of discharge from hospital. Patients in intervention groups received no noticeable benefits in terms of days spent in hospital relative to control-group patients. Nor were any benefits evident in terms of days spent in the coronary-care unit. Intervention patients did, however, score significantly lower on two composite indices of chest pain than did control-group subjects and patients receiving both counseling and education experienced significantly fewer cardiac complications during hospitalization than either the education group or the control group patients. This pattern was also reflected in a measure of state anxiety. Thus, while the results of the study were not quite so encouraging as those reported by Gruen (1975), and the number of patients examined were appreciably smaller, this study once more presents empirical evidence in support of a range of benefits to be gained by early psychological intervention following myocardial infarction.

The mechanisms through which early intervention exerts its influence seem likely to be related in complex ways to the modification of a variety of maladaptive responses to myocardial infarction of the kind discussed in earlier chapters. Gruen (1975), for example, suggested that benefits arising from early psychological intervention came about either because they produced a decrease in the overall level of arousal or because they facilitated the use of active coping resources in the face of crisis. Both of these suggestions ultimately reduce to the notion that rapid intervention decreases cardiovascular activation in the short term and might act to attentuate disproportionate cardiovascular responses to a challenging environment in the long term. As a consequence, feelings of psychological well-being appear to be enhanced and the cardiovascular system as a whole may be given a degree of protection from further damage. Because the myocardium following myocardial infarction is both compromised and vulnerable to the effects of excessive demand (Frankenhaeuser, 1976; Razin, 1982), it is logical to assume that strategies aimed at arousal reduction will decrease the risk of cardiovascular incidents during the acute phase following myocardial infarction. Moreover, the characteristic enhancement of psychological well-being associated with arousal reduction, together perhaps with a decrease in the experience of cardiovascular complications and distress, may produce in the patient a more optimistic attitude toward the future and therefore a greater readiness toward social reintegration and return to work. This approach, which amounts to the modification of abnormal illness behavior early in the patient's illness experience (Byrne et al., 1978), holds considerable promise and would seem to command much greater attention in the future psychological management of the cardiac patient than it has in the past.

3.3   The Post-Hospital Phase

By contrast with the acute phase, the post-hospital phase following myocardial infarction has attracted a useful number of well-conducted studies evaluating the effectiveness of psychological and behavioral intervention. Once more, one might speculate on the reasons for this; however they have probably as much to do with convenience as with scientific rationale. While the patients in the coronary-care unit constitute a captive population for intervention practice and research, the convenience of initiating this intervention, particularly in groups, is clearly greater once the patient has left hospital. Moreover, the real or implied risk of cardiovascular complications which exist during the acute phase decreases by the time of discharge from hospital, as evidenced by the fact that the physician has seen fit to release the patient from continuing medical care. Intervention may, therefore, be initiated with a greater degree of security that a more stable cardiovascular system will not respond adversely to the strategies being used. It has also been suggested that anxiety peaks and depression begins to develop around the time of hospital discharge (Cassem & Hackett, 1971; Byrne, 1979), presenting perhaps an opportune time for the emotional management of the cardiac patient. Finally, the patient's emotional state, together with the recognition of the fact that re-entry into social and family roles and active employment is now a distinct possibility, may act to increase the patient's compliance with the various behavioral strategies involved in post-hospital intervention. It is perhaps not too surprising then, that this phase of the cardiac patient's progress has served as the primary focus for behavioral and psychological intervention.

Thockloth, Ho, Wright, and Seldon (1973) examined the effects on outcome of psychological intervention with 50 randomly selected males who had survived a first myocardial infarction and related this to the clinical cases who were offered only routine medical care. The intervention was offered on an individual basis by an occupational therapist and a social worker and involved regular weekly contact beginning during the final stages of hospitalization and extending over three months after discharge from hospital. The primary emphasis of intervention was on counseling (amounting to short-term psychotherapy) to deal with the resolution of social, emotional, and financial problems following myocardial infarction. A long-term follow-up of all patients demonstrated a range of advantages to be gained from intervention even when it is simply directed at practical issues such as these. While intervention did not result in a more rapid return to work, it was found that a greater number of intervention than control patients returned to work during an ''optimal'' period of time, which the authors defined as two to four months following myocardial infarction. Intervention patients were also more compliant with medical advice and instructions than were control patients, and reported less emotional distress, and in particular depression, during the post-hospital period, than did patients whose only contact was with their medical practitioners. This latter finding is not surprising, as the intervention was specifically aimed at the management of emotional distress and of the psychosocial conditions that might precipitate this. Moreover, intervention patients had the benefit of regular contact with a care giver, while control patients had only spasmodic contact with their medical advisers. Nonetheless, the study supports the value of individual psychotherapy as an aid to rehabilitation following myocardial infarction.

A similar emphasis was taken by Adsett and Bruhn (1968)—however patients (all male) were, in this instance, specifically selected for the fact that they were experiencing substantial psychological problems following myocardial infarction. By contrast with the previous study, however, these patients were treated in a group and their wives received simultaneous group therapy, undertaken separately but organized along similar lines. A control group consisted of six male patients who had survived myocardial infarction and who were matched on demographic characteristics to those in the intervention group but who received nothing other than routine medical care. Intervention involved regular outpatient contacts extending over 10 sessions and concerned with supportive but exploratory psychotherapy aimed at the resolution of specific problems raised by individual patients within the group.

While the therapeutic program appeared to be well accepted by the intervention patients, they experienced little additional advantage relative to control patients either on measures indicating relief from psychological distress or in terms of risk of subsequent cardiac events. Patients with psychological problems who refused to participate in the intervention group (though not control patients) appeared to suffer a higher frequency of subsequent cardiac events. However, the small numbers involved (four) strongly limited the inferences that could be drawn from this.

Bruhn et al. (1971) followed the long-term outcomes of these same patients over several years after psychotherapeutic intervention. This provision appeared to confer no real advantages with regard to long-term relief from psychological distress; however, there was a trend among patients in the intervention group to show rates of long-term survival in excess of those patients in the control group.

The first extensive and controlled study of post-hospital psychological intervention in survivors of myocardial infarction was reported by Ibrahim and his colleagues (Ibrahim, Feldman, Sultz, Staiman, Young, & Dean, 1974). Subjects were both male and female patients between 35 and 65 years of age, who had been admitted to a coronary-care unit with a confirmed myocardial infarction. They were approached shortly after discharge from hospital and the first 12 eligible and consenting patients were assigned to an intervention group. The second 12 patients were assigned to a control group. This procedure was repeated until five intervention and five control groups were achieved. Fifty of the final 70 intervention patients completed the entire course of the intervention program and were followed up, while outcome data were obtained for the entire 60 patients in the control groups.

Patients in the intervention groups were given one-and-a-half hours of group therapy weekly for a total of 50 weeks. The aim of this therapy was to provide an atmosphere in which problems and solutions common to cardiac patients could be shared. The therapists (experienced clinical psychologists) served primarily to encourage exploration of emotion and attitudes surrounding the myocardial infarction. It avoided, as far as possible, any educative role with regard to exercise, diet, and medication. Patients were encouraged to raise these issues with their physicians as the most appropriate providers of such information. While patients appeared comfortable in discussing the relatively pragmatic, concrete issues of resumption of leisure, social activity, and return to active employment, there was an observed tendency among them to redirect discussions away from issues of emotional response and self-exploration of difficulties. Therapists were encouraged to counteract this tendency as far as they were able, though the phenomemon of avoidance of self-disclosure appears to be a common one in studies of psychological intervention following physical illnesses (Blanchard & Miller, 1977).

Patients in the control groups were offered routine follow-up contact with their physicians; however, no attempt was made to provide anything other than normal medical care as indicated by individual patient's conditions. At this level, of course, nothing was denied to the patient by way of intervention which might have been beneficial to recovery and maintenance of health.

At discharge from hospital, both intervention and control patients were found to be closely similar on a quantitative prognostic index of outcome after myocardial infarction (the Peel Index). Follow-up examinations were made on all intervention patients completing the program and all control patients at 6, 12, and 18 months after discharge from hospital. Intervention subjects showed a high level of compliance with the activity of group therapy, though 10 failed to complete the course. While there was no difference between intervention and control patients in rates of rehospitalizations during the follow-up period, the mean duration of rehospitalization for intervention patients was significantly shorter than that for control patients. Though follow-up examinations suggested that intervention patients achieved no greater benefits in terms of reductions of levels of emotional distress and coronary risk factors than those in control groups, the study produced one very important result. That was that, at 18-month follow-up, intervention patients (who had been matched on all important prognostic variables with control patients) showed a 10% lower mortality rate from subsequent myocardial infarction than did their colleagues in the control groups. The importance of this finding is that it demonstrates the long-term survival benefits to be gained by psychological intervention following myocardial infarction. It should be remembered, however, that intervention patients participated in group therapy in a medical setting over the course of 50 weeks, and this may have sensitized them to seek help for perceived cardiac irregularities sooner than the control patients. This may, in time, have conferred on them a distinct survival advantage. By contrast, control patients, who were receiving only routine and irregular medical care, may have been more likely to deny or ignore the first symptoms of subsequent coronary events and, therefore, less likely to seek medical attention for these.

The additional value of this study was that it provided descriptive clinical information on a broad range of issues and difficulties which become evident during psychological intervention with cardiac patients. This material, which has been considered by Ibrahim (1976), provides an informative clinical background for the psychological management of a range of problems emerging after myocardial infarction.

A novel approach to the psychological management of the cardiac patient was reported by Prince and Miranda (1977). This was based on the notion that at least part of the recurrence rate following myocardial infarction could be explained in terms of the experience of a surfeit of distressing life events in the recovery phase, much along the lines of the life events explanations of first epidsodes of myocardial infarction (Byrne & Whyte, 1980) which have been prominent in the recent literature. Thirty seven survivors of a first myocardial infarction were enlisted into the study one week after discharge from hospital. At this point, all patients were interviewed by telephone and a 20 item self-report scale of psychological distress (the General Health Questionnaire of Goldberg, 1972) was administered by a psychologist. All patients were then followed up by telephone at monthly intervals over a period of seven months and the same scale was given at each follow-up point. Whenever a patient scored five or more on the General Health Questionnaire (a common cut-off point indicating a potentially high level of psychological distress) a nurse was notified and she made another telephone call to arrange a home visit. Patients almost always agreed to this.

A retrospective view of the experience reported by Prince and Miranda (1977) identified three primary areas of difficulty for which intervention was indicated. The first related to the simple provision of information concerning myocardial infarction and its medical treatment, and literature was prepared for distribution to assist patients in understanding this process. The second related to difficulties reported in social, economic, and interpersonal areas experienced by patients, and this resulted either in referral to social workers or back to the physician. Finally, some patients required periodic emotional support and reassurance which was provided by the nurse. Occasionally, referral for psychiatric attention was necessary.

There was a strong and significant correlation between levels of emotional and life stress following myocardial infarction and the probability of rehospitalization. Moreover, where intervention was indicated by scores on the General Health Questionnaire but was unable to be initiated for one reason or another, the rates of rehospitalization and subsequent cardiac death were greater than where intervention was either not indicated or was indicated and given. While this study is small and was not designed as a prospective outcome study, its value is that it presents the novel approach of monitoring an individual patient's needs and of offering intervention on this needs basis. As such, it appears to have been both economical and, to the extent that evaluation could take place, effective in reducing both emotional distress and, possibly, further coronary events. While studies of this kind can not identify the active components of therapeutic intervention, they add to the evidence that interventions generally aimed at reducing emotional distress after heart attack can also act to reduce further coronary risk.

An extensive study by Naismith et al (1979) once more focused attention on male patients under 60 years of age who had survived a first myocardial infarction. A consecutive series of such patients were randomly allocated either to intensive intervention or control groups, resulting in 76 in the former and 77 in the latter. The initial contact was made on the third day after hospital admission while the patient was still in the coronary-care unit, and regular contacts with a nurse (and a medical practitioner where necessary) were then initiated over a six-month post-hospital period. Patients were seen individually, both on an outpatient basis and in their own homes, and wives were actively encouraged to participate in the intervention. The intervention procedure was open ended and involved counseling directed toward the achievement of maximum independence and medical advice with regard to secondary preventative measures for myocardial infarction. Both the patient and his wife were educated to understand the nature of the illness and were encouraged during intervention to express any fears and difficulties which they had experienced. Regular follow-up for outcome evaluation was made at six weeks, 12 weeks, and six months after myocardial infarction.

Patients allocated to the control group received routine medical care and printed educational material relating to risk factors for subsequent myocardial infarction. They received no other active rehabilitation but were followed up six months after discharge from hospital to assess their outcome experience.

Patients in the intervention group were substantially more effective in achieving social independence over the follow-up period than were control patients. Moreover, the former group returned to work in a significantly shorter period of time than did the latter group, even though the physical and other demands of the occupations to which they returned were not different. When patients in the intervention group were divided according to their levels of neuroticism (as measured by the Neuroticism Scale of the Eysenck Personality Inventory), it was found that those with high levels of this attribute were more likely than others to achieve benefits from psychological intervention. While this might indicate, paradoxically, that outcome after myocardial infarction is facilitated to an extent by the patient's neurotic state, there was no change over the follow-up period in neuroticism scores for either patient group; a more likely explanation might, therefore, rest with the facilitation of therapeutic compliance among patients with elevated levels of psychological arousal accompanying a neurotic state. Interestingly, the initial severity of the myocardial infarction and the continuing physical symptoms which this produced in some patients had little or no bearing either on psychological or occupational outcomes.

These results add to the encouraging evidence that psychological intervention following myocardial infarction can produce outcome benefits. The point of overriding importance for Naismith and her colleagues appeared to be that psychological intervention can be both open ended and conducted relatively economically using nursing staff as the primary facilitators of behavioral change.

The primary focus of a study by Rahe and his colleagues (Rahe, O'Neil, Hagan, & Arthur, 1975; Rahe, Ward, & Hayes, 1979) was the provision of group therapy in the rehabilitation of survivors of myocardial infarction. In common with most other studies in the area, patients consisted of survivors under the age of 60 years of a first myocardial infarction. Initial intake involved the random allocation of half a consecutive series of admissions to an intervention group and the other half to a control group resulting in equal group sizes of 22 patients each. The early success of the program produced, however, an enthusiasm for the group psychotherapeutic approach among both prospective patients and staff, so that an additional 17 patients who met the admission criteria were allocated to psychological intervention. Both intervention samples and the control sample were matched on a variety of sociodemographic variables and on a quantitative index of the severity of the myocardial infarction. All patients involved in the study were contacted prior to discharge from hospital and those allocated to intervention groups were scheduled to commence these approximately one month after discharge. Groups consisted of approximately four patients and one psychiatrically trained therapist (sometimes with a co-therapist) and involved six sessions of 90 minutes each, held once every two weeks. Patients were expected to attend all six sessions. Spouses were invited to participate in the second session, which covered the role of physical and psychological risk factors in the genesis of coronary heart disease; all other sessions were closed.

Attendance averaged greater than 75%. While there was no adherence to a strict therapeutic program, the six sessions covered the areas of (a) life stress and the onset of myocardial infarction, (b) the contribution of physical and psychological risk factors to coronary heart disease, (c) the coronary-prone behavior pattern, (d) home problems, and (e) problems associated with return to work after heart attack. The major approach to the group sessions was an educational one. Groups were problem oriented and an active discussion of problems encountered by patients was encouraged. Occasionally, specific behavioral prescriptions were given to individual patients in an effort to modify coronary-prone behaviors; however this was the exception rather than the rule and was used only where patients demonstrated a high potential to benefit from such an exercise. Control subjects received no active rehabilitation procedures of a psychological kind but were given routine follow-up medical care.

Follow-up examinations were conducted at intervals of six months, 18 months, 36 months, and 48 months after myocardial infarction. The study demonstrated a range of benefits to be gained from the psychological intervention. A significantly greater number of control subjects than intervention subjects were hospitalized for coronary insufficiency during the first six months of follow-up, though this trend was not maintained over the total four-year follow-up period. Patients in the intervention group did, however, experience significantly fewer re-infarctions over the four-year follow-up period than did patients in the control group. The period between seven and 18 months following myocardial infarction also saw a significantly greater number of coronary artery bypass operations in control patients relative to those involved in group therapy. These benefits to cardiological outcome did not, however, spill over into measures of coronary mortality, and long-term survival rates did not appear to be influenced by psychological intervention. In addition to the apparent cardiovascular benefits to be gained by intervention, patients who participated in group therapy were more likely to return to full-time work during the follow-up period than were control patients. While there was considerable variability in patients' affective status levels (of depression and anxiety) over the course of the follow-up period, psychological intervention appeared to confer no consistent benefit on emotional outcome following myocardial infarction. This is surprising in view of the nature of the intervention (its psychological orientation) and of the accumulating evidence supporting the potential benefits of psychological intervention on affective distress after myocardial infarction. Neither was there a consistent influence of psychological intervention on a variety of physical risk factors (body weight, cigarette smoking, or serum cholesterol) or on the presence of the coronary-prone behavior pattern over the course of intervention.

The importance of this study lies not only in its positive outcomes but also with the fact that its therapeutic elements were not open ended but well specified and clearly described. This imparts the study with replicability and allows for an integration of the intervention strategy into routine clinical practice.

A modest study by Fielding (1980) was the first to specifically address the issue of problem-oriented behavior modification following myocardial infarction. Intervention rested on the assumption that a variety of behaviors commonly observed in response to myocardial infarction, notably anxiety, depression and tension, might act to increase the risk of subsequent cardiac events by producing elevations in levels of psychophysiological arousal. This theme was by no means new and had been raised by others, (Gruen, 1975) as a means of explaining the mechanisms through which psychological intervention produced outcome benefits. Fielding's study was also based, however, on a consistent speculation (Nagle, Gangola, & Picton-Robinson, 1971; Cay et al., 1973) that such outcomes as social integration and return to work were more a function of the emotional and behavioral adjustments which patients made to myocardial infarction than of the severity of the infarction itself.

Ten male patients under 60 years of age and representing a consecutive series of admissions to a coronary-care unit with a diagnosis of first confirmed myocardial infarction were randomly allocated either to an intervention or control group. The five subjects in the intervention group were offered 10 sessions of group intervention each lasting 90 minutes, extending over 10 weeks, and commencing shortly after discharge from hospital. The first hour of each session was devoted to the resolution of emotional difficulties and adjustment problems following myocardial infarction and adopted a problem-solving approach drawing on a variety of behavorial strategies. One session was given over entirely to education regarding the physical mechanisms and risk factors for myocardial infarction and was conducted by a physician. The remaining sessions were conducted by a clinical psychologist. The final half hour of each session was devoted to progressive muscle relaxation training and home relaxation exercises were facilitated by the provision of an audio tape. Patients in the control group were given routine medical care during this 10-week period. Both groups were matched with respect to age, social class, and severity of the myocardial infarction.

Both self-report and psychophysiological assessments of emotional arousal were made on intake into the study and following the 10-week intervention/control period. Intervention subjects showed a significant reduction in muscle tension levels (as measured electromyographically) over the course of therapy and this result was paralleled by self-reported measures of anxiety. No such temporal changes was observed for control subjects. Moreover, a significantly greater number of intervention than control subjects were able to return to work over this 10-week period. No outcome dates were collected on subsequent coronary events.

This study was limited in scope and involved only 10 patients who were followed up over a short period of time. Nonetheless, the encouraging results together with an emphasis on replicable behavioral strategies, make it a potential model for the development of standardized behavioral intervention packages following myocardial infarction.

The trend away from open-ended programs of psychological intervention after myocardial infarction and toward programs using more defined and circumscribed behavioral strategies is exemplified in a study by Langosch, Seer, Brodner, Kallinke, Kulick, and Heim (1982). Patients for this study were male survivors of a first myocardial infarction under the age of 60 years. While these patients had been discharged from hospital, all were at the time of the study inpatients in a cardiac rehabilitation center. Participation was voluntary and, in contrast to other studies, approximately 40% of patients were reluctant to take part in any psychological program of rehabilitation. The authors draw on their clinical experience to explain this phenomenon as being consistent with a wariness among postinfarction patients toward psychotherapy in that particular society (West Germany). This apparent effect of culture or of societal values on acceptance of one approach to intervention may have important clinical implications, not just when comparing approaches between cultures but also when dealing with patients from different cultural groups within one clinical setting.

The study compared two strategies of behavioral management, the first involving a stress-management program and the second focusing specifically on progressive muscle relaxation. Participation in these two groups was according to personal preference, with the former group attracting 32 patients, the latter 28. A random allocation procedure resulted in a further 30 subjects being assigned to a control group. Consistent with previous studies, the patients in these three groups were matched with respect to age, social class, and indices of the severity of myocardial infarction.

Intervention was conducted in groups and was intensively applied. It consisted of eight sessions, each lasting one hour and extending over the entire two-week period of the patient's rehabilitation hospitalization. Both intervention groups emphasized learned sensitivity so as to recognize early cues of tension and on doing so, to engage in coping behaviors to reduce the consequent arousal. A distinct sequence of intervention steps was followed by both groups. The self-management program focused on four major areas of activity. These were, in order; (a) an emphasis on the harmful effects of achievement-oriented behavior on coronary risk factors and the compromised myocardium, (b) training in the discrimination and subsequent modification of self-statements relating to achievement orientation and other cognitions resulting in arousal, by means of the several techniques of thought stopping, the use of positive self-statements incompatible with anxiety and arousal, and the inhibition of unrealistic self-demands concerning occupational success, (c) facilitation of assertive behavior, particularly with regard to colleagues and superiors in the occupational situation, once more using cognitive techniques to enhance positive self-statements but also involving role play and covert rehearsal, and (d) discrimination training in order to become more sensitive to cues for stress, and the modification of this state when it was perceived. These sessions were reinforced by a treatment manual written specifically for the study and given serially to patients following each section of the program. It should be noted that the behavioral strategies utilized in this program emphasized a cognitive approach to reduce both psycho-physiological arousal and coronary-prone behaviors. This approach is reminiscent of now-popular stress management program (Meichenbaum, 1977) that have been found effective in the treatment of both affective distress (typically anxiety states) and states of psychophysiological disturbance.

The relaxation group followed a program involving a modified version of Jacobson's progressive muscle relaxation which went on to emphasize the use of regular breathing exercises as an aid to relaxation and was followed by autogenic training exercises centered on perceptions of "heaviness and "warmth," at the termination of the relaxation exercises and were encouraged to generalize these to situations outside the rehabilitation hospital. Patients in the control group received routine medical care but no direct psychological intervention.

Information on cardiological status, socioeconomic class, and a variety of aspects of present emotional state were collected prior to intervention and immediately following the intervention program. A six-month follow-up of patients discharged from the rehabilitation hospital was also undertaken to assess outcome. No measure of either cariological status or of social, demographic, or occupational variables distinguished between either of the two intervention groups, or the control group, on intake into the study. At the termination of the program, patients in the relaxation group reported a significantly reduced frequency of cardiac complications relative to patients in either the stress management or control groups. By contrast, patients in the self-management group reported decreased work stress and increased assertiveness in the occupational situation relative to both the other groups. At six-month follow-up, both intervention groups appeared to have an advantage in terms of return to work, relative to the control group, however patients in the stress management group experienced significantly less difficulty in this respect than did patients in the relaxation group. Advantages which were manifest in terms of decreases in symptoms of cardiac distress and increases in levels of social and emotional adjustment, evident at the termination of program, appeared by and large to be maintained over the follow-up period, regardless of intervention group.

While acknowledging the limitations of the study (and by contrast with some other work, the relatively large sample sizes together with the controlled nature of the project and the detailed specification of therapeutic interventions make it a very credible study) Langosch and his colleagues concluded that both treatment procedures produced improvements in psychological and occupational adjustment not evident in the control group. Benefits were most evident in terms of modifications of assertive and achievement-oriented behavior and social anxiety and those modifications which were evident also appeared to be maintained over time. Moreover, there was evidence that the coping skills learned during intervention generalized to everyday life situations and were maintained following the termination of the intervention program.

The effects of behavioral self-management and relaxation were by no means identical. Behavioral self-management appeared to persuade patients that they were able to invoke the use of coping mechanisms in the face of stressful life experiences following discharge from hospital. This program acted to improve patient's abilities to recognize and discriminate aspects of a stressful environmental situation as cues emerged from it, and to initiate activity from a repertoire of coping mechanisms in order to deal with this stress. The primary recommendation arising from the study is that the combination of behavioral self-management and relaxation into an interventive package should serve to enlarge the patient's coping repertoire and improve discrimination abilities in the face of life stress so as to enhance capacity for self-control over stressful conditions in daily life.

A recent study by VanDixhoorn, De Loos, and Duivenvoorden (1983) looked specifically at the effects of progressive muscle relaxation training on outcomes following myocardial infarction. The rationale underlying this specific focus rested on three assumptions: (a) relaxation is a technique effective at a psychophysiological level both in reducing arousal and promoting a sense of psychological well-being, (b) it provides the individual with direct feedback and, therefore, a sensitivity to adequately estimate present emotional and physical states, and (c) it can be taught and practiced conveniently in most rehabilitation settings after only a small amount of training.

Subjects were drawn from patients applying to join a coronary rehabilitation program who satisfied the criteria that they had suffered a well-documented myocardial infarction, were physically able to join a program involving exercise, and had been discharged from hospital for a period of less than three weeks. All subjects were assessed for subjective perceptions of cardiac symptoms, immediate psychological state, sleep quality, and unpleasant bodily experiences. Following this, they were randomly assigned to one of two groups, the first involving relaxation training and the second being a control group and focusing only on exercise retraining. The relaxation procedure involved the use of electromyographic biofeedback from the frontalis muscle, together with instructions and guidance about diaphragmatic breathing. Patients were also given instructions for passive relaxation so that they could generalize the procedure to situations outside the clinic. Relaxation instructions were given individually, in sessions averaging one hour's duration occurring weekly over six weeks. Patients in this group were also given exercise retraining using a standard bicycle ergometer, adjusted to allow peak loads of 80% of maximal heart rate. Patients in the control group received only exercise retraining and were placed on a five-week program of daily training on the bicycle ergometer, once more directed toward the attainment of peak loads of 80% of maximal heart rate. Exercise retraining was accomplished in groups of four patients. A repeat evaluation of all intake variables was given to all patients immediately upon termination of the intervention procedures.

Relaxation training conferred no outcome benefits additional to exercise retraining on measures of anxiety, sleep quality, or somatic stress. Patients in the relaxation group did, however, report significantly higher scores on a scale of subjective well-being and significantly lower scores on a scale reflecting perceived invalidity than did subjects in the exercise-only group. The strength of these differences led the authors to conclude that the addition of relaxation training made a positive and substantial contribution to the well-being of patients following myocardial infarction. Regrettably, the outcome measures were restricted to those of subjective experience immediately upon termination of the intervention program, and follow-up was not undertaken for a sufficiently long period of time to examine the influence of relaxation training on measures of occupational rehabilitation and subsequent coronary morbidity and mortality. The short-term benefits of this program seem, nonetheless, to be very worthwhile and long-term studies of the intervention strategies would appear to be indicated.

4.   IMPLICATIONS FOR CLINICAL PRACTICE

The collective impression to be distilled from the range of reports and empirical studies reviewed in this chapter encourages the use of psychological and behavioral strategies for intervention following myocardial infarction. While the studies vary widely, both in sophistication of design and in the theoretical orientations of intervention strategies, the evidence as a whole consistently supports the conclusion that recovery and rehabilitation after myocardial infarction may be facilitated by the provision of psychological assistance. The bulk of demonstrated outcome benefits has centered either on reductions in levels of psychological distress and enhancement of feelings of psychological and physical well-being or on the ease and rapidity of return to work. This is not surprising, as the focus of intervention has frequently been to counteract the emotional distress following myocardial infarction, and it has now been amply demonstrated that return to work is as much a function of an individual's subjective feelings of well-being as it is of the physical severity of the myocardial infarction. However, in a small number of studies where sample sizes and follow-up periods were sufficiently large to allow such outcome benefits to emerge, there was encouraging evidence that appropriate psychological management following myocardial infarction may act to confer long-term cardiac stability and survival benefits on the survivor of myocardial infarction.

In extrapolating from these data to guidelines for clinical practice, a series of distinct and related issues stand out for comment. These issues fall into the following categories and must be seen as central to the selection of appropriate intervention strategies or the compilation of packages.

4.1   Acute versus Outpatient Intervention

The practical arguments for and against the provision of psychological intervention either in the coronary-care unit or outpatient settings are discussed in Sections 3.2 and 3.3. There is as yet too little information on the efficacy of coronary-care-unit intervention to allow a useful comparison to be made, and the present evidence indicates no overall superiority of one over the other. Razin (1982) cites a number of studies, however, which recommend the early initiation of psychological intervention. Cassem and Hackett (1973) imply, for example, that the resolution of emotional distress during the very early stages of recovery from myocardial infarction may circumvent difficulties which might otherwise arise during later stages of recovery and rehabilitation. Moreover, the well designed and executed study by Gruen (1975) presents persuasive evidence of the outcome benefits which might accrue from rapid intervention following hospitalization. All this is consistent with the growing medical opinion that early mobilization of the patient is preferable to long periods of bed rest. Consideration should, therefore, be given to the commencement, at least, of psychological intervention in the acute phase after myocardial infarction wherever practical and organizational considerations allow this.

4.2   Individual versus Group Intervention

A roughly equal number of studies have involved intervention with individuals and in groups, though there has been no systematic comparison of these two approaches. Practical considerations may well be a deciding factor. It is clearly difficult to undertake group work with patients still in intensive medical care. However, group intervention may be the most cost-effective means of management after discharge from hospital. There is some evidence (Cassem & Hackett, 1971) that at least one peak of emotional distress occurs in the early days following myocardial infarction, at a point where the compromized myocardium is perhaps most vulnerable to physiological instability, and there is further evidence (Ibrahim et al., 1974; Blanchard & Miller, 1977) the groups of cardiac patients, once discharged from hospital, are reluctant to explore feelings and attitudes and are more comfortable with concrete, problem-oriented, and educational experiences. It is possible then, that individual intervention provides the most favorable setting where the focus of intervention is on the resolution of presently experienced emotional distress. On the other hand, group management may offer two distinct therapeutic advantages. The first has to do with the challenge of denial which is so frequently present following myocardial infarction (Byrne et al., 1979). Patients may be less inclined to cling to the defence of denial in a situation where they are confronted with a group of other patients, all of whom have sustained a myocardial infarction and where their own situation no longer appears so unique and threatening. Secondly, where specific behavioral strategies such as role play and behavioral rehearsal are used (Langosch et al., 1982) the availability of a group may facilitate the rehearsal of these strategies and, therefore, strengthen their learning.

4.3   Spouse Involvement

While some studies have involved the patient's spouse in a limited number of intervention sessions (Rahe et al., 1979; Naismith et al., 1979) or have arranged parallel groups for spouses (Adsett & Bruhn, 1968), the majority of intervention trials have not offered any role whatsoever to this important and significant other person. There is very clear evidence (Finlayson & McEwen, 1977) that the spouse forms a crucial variable in the patient's recovery and rehabilitation. There is also evidence (Byrne, 1979) that patient uncertainty and anxiety following myocardial infarction can generate reciprocal uncertainty and anxiety in the spouse (Mayou et al., 1978b). Razin (1982) emphasizes the need for the mobilization of social supports following myocardial infarction, and the role of the spouse is self-evident in this respect. Therefore, while the issue may ultimately reduce to one of patient preference, the evidence presents a persuasive case for the involvement for the spouse in every possible stage of the intervention process.

4.4   Intensity and Duration of Intervention

Once more, there has been wise variation between studies both in the intensity of therapeutic offerings and in the length of time over which these have extended. The modal number of intervention sessions would appear to be one per week, although in acute inpatient interventions at the individual level, daily contact has not been uncommon. The majority of programs favor a time-limited approach involving some weeks or at most some months of intervention, while at least one program, that undertaken by Ibrahim and his colleagues, extended over a whole year after myocardial infarction. At this level, one must obviously question the cost effectiveness of intervention and of the possibility of reinforcing dependence among patients, both on therapists and on the group. Moreover, in view of the evidence on attrition from intervention programs (Ibrahim et al., 1974), one must question whether patients surviving a myocardial infarction will maintain a sufficient commitment to long-term intervention. Therefore, while there is no systematic evidence on the relative value of short- versus long-term programs, the practical considerations would appear to recommend a time-limited procedure.

4.5   Undirected versus Direct Focus Programs

Some intervention programs, notably the early ones, offered relatively open-ended therapy with few specific goals other than the resolution of emotional distress in the face of myocardial infarction, while other programs have been oriented toward the resolution of specific problems which relate hypothetically to outcomes, satisfactory or otherwise, after myocardial infarction. Other programs will have focused on quite specific problem behaviors—for example, poor compliance—in a relatively small number of identified subjects. Some open-ended programs—for example, that reported by Ibrahim and his colleagues—have been characterized by a degree of success; however more rigorous evaluation procedures have generally been attached to those programs, involving a detailed specification of the elements of intervention and a clear statement of the relationships which these might bear to mechanisms of outcome. In this respect, intervention programs which offer a detailed specification of the behavioral strategies for use and an explanation of the rationale underlying their choice, which are by implication also time limited and problem oriented, would seem to offer some advantage over programs in which neither the active elements nor the time course are well specified.

4.6 Relaxation Training

An increasing number of programs (Langosch et al., 1982; Van Dixhoorn et al, 1983) have recently advocated the use of progressive muscle relaxation techniques in psychological intervention after myocardial infarction. The rationale underlying this has to do with the protective influence which arousal-lowering procedures may have on a compromised myocardium. There is now good, direct physiological evidence (Davidson et al., 1979) that deep muscle relaxation may act to lower the overall cardiac workload of patients recovering from myocardial infarction. There seems good reason, therefore, to include deep muscle relaxation as a component of behavioral management following myocardial infarction.

4.7 Patient Education

A consistent theme in the available literature relates to the necessity of education. The provision of simple but direct information about myocardial infarction and its causes and consequences, both to patients and their spouses, can be seen as an element in almost every study of psychological intervention. There are two direct reasons for this. One has to do with the assumption that patients, given specific information about the risks of myocardial infarction, will so modify their own behaviors as to reduce these risks and, therefore, reduce the potential for further cardiac events. The second concerns the notion that a failure to provide this information will produce potentially damaging and maladaptive levels of anxiety, both in patients and their spouses, and that the inclusion of an education phase in intervention will act to circumvent this particular source of postmyocardial infarction distress. The consistency with which education has been used in intervention, together with the reasons underlying it, recommend its continued use in programs of psychological intervention.

4.8 Intervention Packages

There has been some debate (Razin, 1982) as to the relative merits of single-focus intervention programs or those employing a combination of strategies within an intervention package. While a small number of single-focus programs, for example that of Van Dixhoorn et al. (1983), have shown themselves to be useful, these assume that the psychological difficulties predisposing patients to unsatisfactory outcomes are identical across all patients. This is clearly not the case. Nor is it likely that patients will be subject to one specific behavior predisposing to an unsatisfactory outcome. The consensus, therefore, seems to be that of a package of intervention strategies carefully chosen and related to one another by a coherent theoretical framework. This offers advantages in excess of outcome benefits to be gained from single-focus procedures.

4.9   Methodological Cautions

The empirical studies reviewed in this chapter have varied widely in their methodological rigor. While sample sizes for some studies have been respectable, others have used regrettably small numbers of patients; the generality of inferences to be drawn from the results is, therefore, somewhat limited. Follow-up times, too, have frequently been truncated, so that the periods of time available to allow the development of measurable rates of morbidity and mortality from subsequent myocardial infarction have been insufficient. Indeed, in some studies, outcome success has been measured only at termination of the program and such a procedure as this may lead to falsely encouraging results. Attrition rates from intervention groups vary from one study to another; however they remain unacceptably high. Because little is known of the differential dropout rate of successful or unsuccessful patients in intervention programs, the generality of the data is further limited. Outcome measures too, raise some concern. While some studies, particularly those with sufficiently large sample sizes and long follow-up periods, have measured the effects of intervention on morbidity and mortality from subsequent myocardial infarction, others have focused their attention only on rates of return to work measures of psychosocial adaptation or subjective impressions of emotional well-being. While this latter group of outcomes is clearly important and frequently neglected in traditional studies (Byrne, 1982), the need for more ambitious studies to confirm the contribution of psychological and behavioral management to long-term survival clearly exists. Finally, studies vary in the extent to which they have described the intervention programs used. Descriptions range from vague references to supportive group psychotherapy through to detailed prescriptions of specific behavioral strategies; and while there appears to be a temporal trend from open-ended psychological programs to circumscribed packages of well-described behavioral strategies, there is clearly a need in further work for an adequate description of procedures used so as to allow for their replication both as a research exercise and in clinical practice.

CHAPTER 6

The Behavioral Management of Coronary Risk Factors After Myocardial Infarction

1. THE NEED FOR RISK FACTOR MANAGEMENT

The evidence summarized in the first chapter has firmly established that clinical episodes of myocardial infarction can be predicted by the presence of one or more of a set of standard and accepted risk factors reflecting physiological, metabolic, and behavioral processes. Reference to any of the major epidemiological studies of coronary risk will confirm the breadth of risk factors which have been implicated in the genesis of coronary heart disease; however it is generally agreed that the bulk of outcome variance in prospective studies of the incidence of myocardial infarction can be explained by the presence or absence of the three major risk factors of hypertension, elevated levels of cholesterol in the blood, and cigarette smoking. (The role of the Type A Behavior Pattern constitutes a particular case for consideration and will be dealt with in the following chapter.) There is also some epidemiological support for the view that deliberate steps aimed at the reduction of coronary risk factors, whether focused on one simple risk or a collection, can result in a decrease in the risk of myocardial infarction (Kornitzer, De Backer, Dramaix, Kittel, Thilly, Graffar, & Vuylsteek, 1983; the Multiple Risk Factor Intervention Trial, 1976).

The mediation of risk associated with these factors clearly acts by means of complex pathophysiological mechanisms, the nature of which are sometimes obscure and certainly beyond the scope of this work. The risk factors themselves can not be viewed simply as biological phenomena, since this would mask the role which behavior plays, both in their appearance and magnitude. This is seen most strongly with cigarette smoking, where individual behavior is simply responsible for the existence of the risk factor, though there is now very strong evidence to implicate behavioral and psychological states in the regulation and elevation of blood pressure. The relevance of this to the management of the cardiac patient lies directly with the potential for the behavioral control of these risk factors.

Because the cardiovascular system can be severely compromised by the occurrence of a first myocardial infarction, the epidemiological evidence on the contribution of risk factors to recurrent events of the illness is somewhat more contentious. A number of studies (Jenkins et al., 1975; Leeder et al., 1983; Martin et al., 1983) suggest that the persistence of at least some risk factors over time places the survivor of a first myocardial infarction at a measurably elevated risk of a recurrent event. For this reason, prescriptive advice given to survivors of myocardial infarction by their physicians on discharge from hospital will frequently involve cessation of cigarette smoking among smokers. Treatment of hypertension, where this is evident, is most usually undertaken by means of pharmacological therapy. In spite of both the prospective data and the commonly documented activities of physicians, however, there is only limited epidemiological evidence that the systematic control of traditional risk factors following myocardial infarction produces noticeable outcome benefits in terms of increased survival rates and reduced morbidity rates (Wilhelmsen et al., 1982). It may be argued that a compromised cardiovascular system following myocardial infarction adds so many unknowns to the prediction of outcomes as to preclude an uncontaminated and controlled study of the contribution of risk factors. Nonetheless, the attempted medical management of risk factors is routinely practiced following myocardial infarction and the role of behavioral strategies in this process is an increasingly important one.

It is not the purpose of this chapter to establish the superiority of behavioral strategies over medical management in the control of risk factors, though the evidence would indicate that behavioral control has much to offer in an area where the physiological risk is mediated by individual behaviors. Rather, the chapter aims to selectively review the evidence on the behavioral control of the risk factors of hypertension and cigarette smoking. This review will be deliberately brief, as a very large literature already exists to document these areas. Moreover, the bulk of evidence will be taken from studies involving persons with no evidence of clinical coronary heart disease. This is largely because the evidence from survivors of myocardial infarction is somewhat sparse, though there is no reason to believe that evidence of the former kind will be invalidated by the occurrence of myocardial infarction. With this in mind, however, it is possible that patients with coronary heart disease may have particular needs which must be met or particular cautions which must be adhered to; and where these arise they will be spelled out in detail.

While dietary control is often prescribed to control both weight and blood fat levels after heart attack, data on the behavioral management of eating will not be considered. This is firstly because material on the selective control of dietary intake is limited in scope, and, secondly, because the data on dietary regulation of blood fats is contentious.

2.   THE BEHAVIORAL MANAGEMENT OF BLOOD PRESSURE

The clinical and experimental evidence relating patterns of behavior and emotional states to elevations of both systolic and diastolic blood pressure is now sufficiently large and sufficiently persuasive to establish beyond reasonable doubt the psychological contributions to hypertension (Shapiro & Goldstein, 1983). This evidence lays the theoretical foundations for the nonpharmacological control of blood pressure, and a considerable body of literature has accumulated to support the contention that blood pressure can be substantially reduced by means of behavioral or psychological manipulations. A number of recent reviews of this literature have, however, produced somewhat guarded conclusions as to the durability of these changes and, therefore, long-term clinical significance of the behavioral control of blood pressure. The implications of this for clinical practice must be carefully considered.

The evidence supporting the notion that blood pressure can be effectively reduced by means of behavioral and psychological treatments can be roughly categorized under the headings of supportive psychotherapy, relaxation therapy, meditation techniques, biofeedback strategies, and composite procedures. This framework, while clearly not dealing with mutually exclusive categories, provides a convenient structure for a selective overview of the evidence.

2.1   Supportive Psychotherapy

While supportive psychotherapy delivered in line with a range of theoretical stances has been shown to exert a generalized effect on levels of autonomic arousal, with a concomitant reduction in subjectively experienced affective distress, and while the use of supportive psychotherapy as a treatment for psychosomatic symptoms has a long history (Lipowski, Lipsitt, & Whybrow, 1977), the direct treatment of hypertension using psychotherapeutic strategies has been only sparsely reported. Two systematic studies employing interventions organized along psychoanalytic lines (Reiser, Brust, & Ferris, 1951; Moses, Daniels, & Nickerson, 1956) were able to demonstrate quite appreciable falls in blood pressure over the course of psychotherapy in patients suffering from essential hypertension. This evidence is, however, not recent, and studies of psychodynamically oriented psychotherapy for the treatment of psychosomatic symptoms do not appear to have been in favor in the past three decades. Moreover, as Whyte (1983) has pointed out, formal psychotherapy is expensive and time consuming and should be considered for hypertensive patients only where frank psychiatric symptoms dominate the presenting problems.

2.2   Relaxation Techniques

The achievement of deep muscle relaxation either by active Jacobsonian techniques or more passive procedures using mental imagery is one of the most widely used behavioral strategies for the control of blood pressure. As such, it has accumulated a considerable body of supportive evidence (Frumkin, Nathan, Prout & Cohen, 1978; Seer, 1979; Wadden, 1984).

Studies over the past decade have been relatively consistent in the demonstration that relaxation techniques can lower blood pressure in patients with mild to moderate essential hypertension by between 5 and 10 mm/Hg, as least under laboratory conditions or where regular home practice is maintained. Baili (1979) found that systematic therapy produced significantly greater falls in blood pressure than did either supportive psychotherapy or an attention control group involving pseudoelectromyographic biofeedback. Moreover, these changes were maintained over a relatively long follow-up period. The usefulness of relaxation therapy in reducing blood pressure in the short term was mirrored by the results of Taylor, Farquhar, Nelson, and Agras (1977) employing similar procedures, and the superiority of relaxation therapy over supportive psychotherapy was also evident in this study. This distinction did not hold over time, however, though it is unclear whether patients treated with relaxation therapy exhibited subsequent increases in blood pressure over the follow-up period or whether patients treated with supportive psychotherapy went on to experience reductions in blood pressure over this period.

Relaxation therapy has certainly been found to lower blood pressure significantly in excess of that obtained with no treatment control groups (Jorgensen, Houston, & Zuranski, 1981; Southam, Agras, Taylor, & Kraemer, 1982). Moreover, relaxation therapy has been shown to produce greater reductions in blood pressure than graded programs of mild exercise (Luborsky et al., 1982).

Evidence such as this confirms the opinion of Blanchard and Miller (1977) that the use of relaxation therapy can produce clinically significant reductions in blood pressure among hypertensive patients. Indeed, the majority of recent reviews of the area (Frumkin et al., 1978; Seer, 1979) carry the same favorable evaluation of relaxation therapy as a means of reducing blood pressure. This evaluation must, however, be qualified in at least three respects. Firstly, Wadden (1984) has questioned the specificity of the relaxation effect on blood pressure and raised instead the possibility that a positive treatment expectancy along the lines of Bandura's self-efficacy notion (Bandura, 1978) is more likely to account for the apparently widespread success of relaxation therapy in the reduction of blood pressure. Secondly, while some studies support the maintenance of the blood pressure reduction over time, particularly where relaxation therapy is continued outside the treatment setting (Blanchard & Miller, 1977; Engel, Glasgow, & Gaarder, 1983), there is continuing doubt as to the long-term persistence of the treatment outcome outside the treatment situation or in the absence of regular (daily) practice of the relaxation techniques (Blanchard & Miller, 1977). Finally, a number of large and systematic studies comparing the effects of relaxation therapy and antihypertensive medication have failed to confirm the consistent superiority of the former over the latter (Goldstein, Shapiro, Thananopavarn, & Sambhi, 1982; Luborsky et al., 1982; Whyte, 1983).

In this last respect, Andrews, McMahon, Austin, & Byrne (1982) carefully reviewed the results of 37 methodologically credible studies of the nonpharmacological treatment of hypertension and compared these with the results of six outcome studies of antihypertensive medication, three of which involved in excess of 2,000 patients each. The comparative process was undertaken by means of the technique of meta-analysis, where the observed magnitude of a treatment effect is standardized by the variance of the control group. This process revealed that the greatest lowering of blood pressure could be achieved by means of antihypertensive medication. And while relaxation therapy or other procedures based on the learned control of autonomic functioning produced appreciable reductions of blood pressure, these did not match, either in magnitude or persistence, those found in the major drug trials.

The autonomic effects of relaxation therapy on cardiovascular activity would seem to be similar to those resulting from antihypertensive medication (Davidson et al., 1979). Moreover, as both Blanchard and Miller (1977) and Andrews et al. (1982) have pointed out, the potentially unpleasant side effects of antihypertensive medication may militate against its long-term use and against compliance behaviour among patients. Whereas the neutral or even positive side effects of relaxation therapy may actually enhance compliance with treatment and, therefore, produce more long-lasting reductions in blood pressure (Blanchard & Miller, 1977). Engel et al. (1983) have, in fact, suggested a combination of medication and behavioral control in a "stepped care" program as the most effective means of reducing blood pressure.

The consensus would still seem to favour the effectiveness of relaxation therapy in blood-pressure reduction, either as a main treatment or as an adjunct to antihypertensive medication. The relative simplicity of relaxation, together with the evidence in support of its usefulness, would continue to indicate it as a front-line procedure in the control of blood pressure.

2.3   Biofeedback

Following the seminal work of Miller on the learned control of blood pressure (Miller, 1975), the most comprehensive set of studies on the biofeedback-assisted regulation of blood pressure has been conducted by Shapiro and his colleagues. A good account of biofeedback and blood-pressure control in subjects with normal blood pressure has been provided by Shapiro and Surwit (1979), and this interesting though clinically peripheral literature will not be dealt with in the present chapter. In general, it has been found that direct blood pressure biofeedback allows reductions in blood pressure of up to 20 mm/Hg in experimental subjects relative to untreated controls (Frumkin et al., 1978), though baseline blood pressure levels appear to be re-established rapidly after termination of the biofeedback training.

Studies of the effectiveness of blood-pressure biofeedback with hypertensive patients have had a mixed success. A number of reports (Blanchard, Young, & Haynes, 1975; Elder & Eustis, 1975; Kristt & Engel, 1975) have all demonstrated the effectiveness of direct blood pressure biofeedback in patients suffering mild to moderate levels of hypertension, with decreases in systolic blood pressure averaging 20 mm/Hg and decreases in diastolic blood pressure averaging 7 mm/Hg. Moreover, follow-up of these patients indicates that blood pressure reductions can be maintained over a time span of between one and three months. Engel et al. (1983) showed that biofeedback of systolic blood pressure in patients with essential hypertension was superior to relaxation therapy alone. When a combination of treatments was given, patients receiving systolic blood pressure biofeedback followed by relaxation training were able to lower their blood pressure significantly greater than patients in whom the reverse order of intervention strategies was administered. Blood pressure reductions attributable to systolic blood pressure biofeedback were maintained over at least nine months of follow-up.

By contrast, a number of equally well-conducted studies of blood-pressure biofeedback have produced rather less encouraging results. Schwartz and Shapiro (1973) found that feedback of diastolic blood pressure given over 15 daily sessions produced no overall blood-pressure change in six out of seven patients with mild essential hypertension, though one patient was able to demonstrate a reduction in diastolic blood pressure of 14 mm/Hg. Similar findings were reported by Frankel, Patel, & Horwitz (1977) for a sample of 22 patients with essential hypertension. In their meta-analysis of the effect sizes of nonpharmacologic treatments of hypertension, Andrews et al. (1982) examined outcomes from eight studies of the use of blood-pressure biofeedback in the treatment of essential hyptertension and concluded that this treatment modality was not only inferior in effectiveness to relaxation or pharmacological means of blood-pressure control but produced reductions in blood pressure not significantly different to those emerging from placebo conditions. This conclusion is reflected in the reviews of others (Blanchard & Miller, 1977; Frumkin et al., 1978; Whyte, 1983). It would seem, therefore, that the initial promise of direct blood-pressure biofeedback for the control of essential hypertension emerging from early studies of hypertensives or experimental studies of normo-tensive subjects has not been fulfilled in later investigations.

It is worth noting that two modalities of biofeedback other than that of direct blood pressure have been employed with limited success in the reduction of blood pressure. Surwit, Shapiro, and Good (1978) compared the effects of blood-pressure biofeedback, feedback of integrated forearm and frontalis muscle electromyographic activity, and a meditation-based relaxation procedure in the treatment of borderline essential hypertension. Electromyographic biofeedback proved to be as effective in reducing blood pressure as direct feedback of blood pressure or meditation mediated relaxation, though this reduction in blood pressure was not maintained over a one-year follow-up period. Biofeedback of electrodermal reactivity as an index of autonomic arousal has also been used to reduce blood pressure (Patel, 1975; Patel, Marmot, & Terry, 1981). In both instances, electrodermal biofeedback was superior to a meditation-based relaxation procedure in reducing both systolic and diastolic blood pressure and these changes were maintained over the course of an eight- to 12-month follow-up period.

The collective equivocality of results from studies using biofeedback leaves some doubt as to its clinical usefulness in the management of the cardiac patient. It has been suggested (Frumkin et al., 1978) that reductions in diastolic blood pressure are more clinically important than changes in systolic blood pressure, since the former are more closely related to cardiovascular morbidity. Shapiro. Mainardi, and Surwit (1977) claimed, however, that biofeedback techniques to reduce abnormally high levels of diastolic blood pressure in patients with hypertension were of only limited usefulness. Thus, even though there is some evidence that biofeedback training for the reduction of systolic blood pressure also results in decreases in diastolic blood pressure (Frumkin et al., 1978) the potential for blood-pressure biofeedback to reduce the risk of hypertension-related morbidity in the cardiac patient would seem to require further classification.

The one area of promise for biofeedback may lie with its use in combination with other forms of the behavioral control of hypertension. Both Seer (1979), and Engel et al. (1983) have indicated that a combination of blood-pressure biofeedback with relaxation techniques may produce reductions in blood pressure in excess of those gained by the use of blood-pressure biofeedback alone. However, while these results are encouraging, the reliance of blood-pressure biofeedback on sophisticated equipment, the doubts which some hold as to the reliability of blood-pressure measures, and their presentation in the form of feedback (Frumkin et al., 1978) and the continually equivocal nature of both outcome and comparative studies of blood-pressure biofeedback do not recommend it as the treatment of choice for the cardiac patient with persistent hypertension.

2.4 Meditation

The physiological effects of meditation, whether by passive imagery or assisted by the use of mantra, are now well documented. There is persuasive evidence that at least in some settings and in some individuals, meditation can produce quite profound reductions in levels of autonomic arousal (Green & Green, 1977). It is not surprising, therefore, that meditation techniques have been studied in the search for an effective nonpharmacological control of blood pressure.

The bulk of research on meditation and its blood-pressure-lowering effects has come from the laboratory of Benson and his colleagues. Benson, Rosner, and Marzetta (1973) showed that daily practice of transcendental meditation over two weeks succeeded in producing significant reductions in systolic but not diastolic blood pressure relative to base-line measures in a sample of 30 patients being treated for essential hypertension. A nine-week follow-up indicated the persistence of the therapeutic effect, so long as the meditation procedure was continued. This same group (Benson et al., 1974a, 1974b) were able to repeat these findings in two further studies and to establish the maintenance of blood-pressure reductions over a period of at least 25 weeks. The studies were, however, of a single group outcome design; and in the absence of a control group, there is no evidence as to whether meditation was superior, either to other means of blood-pressure control or to placebo.

In a controlled study, Stone and De Leo (1976) were able to demonstrate significant decreases in both systolic and diastolic blood pressure in a group of hypertensive patients practicing a relaxation technique relative to a small group of control patients who, by contrast, demonstrated no reduction in blood pressure over time. However, Pollack, Weber, and Case (1977) were unable to show any effective reductions in either systolic or diastolic blood pressure in a group of 20 hypertensive patients regularly practicing a transcendental meditation technique. While systolic blood pressure did decline in the first three months of treatment, these reductions were not maintained over time and, at the end of the study, blood-pressure levels were not appreciably idfferent from base line. Nor were Surwit, Shapiro, and Good (1978) able to demonstrate the superiority of a meditation technique over blood pressure or electromyographic biofeedback in the regulation of blood pressure in essential hypertensives.

The evidence indicating meditation procedures as an effective control of blood pressure must, therefore, be treated with some caution. Meta-analytic review of the literature undertaken by Andrews et al. (1982) suggests that, on balance, meditation techniques were as effective as muscle-relaxation techniques in the control of blood pressure but marginally inferior to antihypertensive medication. Two qualifications at least must, however, be attached to this conclusion. The first concerns the distinction between meditation and other relaxation techniques. It is likely that the physiological consequences of both relaxation and meditation are very similar (Green & Green, 1977) and it may be more convenient in clinical practice to apply a relaxation procedure based on Jacobsonian muscle-relaxation exercises than to rely on the more intricate and perhaps more demanding procedures of meditation in whatever form they take. Secondly, the evaluative studies of meditation appear to have relied largely on single group outcome designs, with very few studies employing control groups. This limits the inferences that may be drawn from the data, and therefore constrains the enthusiasm which was initially held for the use of meditation in the control of blood pressure. Meditation may yet have a place in clinical practice for those who accept the spiritual principles upon which it is based. The evidence would not, however, recommend it as the principal nonpharmacological strategy for the management of hypertension in the survivor of heart attack.

2.5 Overview

The weight of evidence would appear to favor simple Jacobsonian relaxation procedures as the first nonpharmacological treatment of choice in the regulation of high blood pressure among cardiac patients. Its efficacy has been consistently demonstrated in well-controlled outcome studies, its use supported by recent critical reviews (Frumkin et al., 1978; Seer, 1979; Whyte, 1983). While the evidence does not allow claims for the superiority of relaxation or other behavioral procedures over antihypertensive medication in the treatment of high blood pressure, the potential disadvantages of side effects arising from medication together with the influence which these might have on compliance (Blanchard & Miller, 1977) foreshadow a continued need for the use of nonpharmacological treatments at least as an adjunct to medication in the control of high blood pressure.

3. THE BEHAVIORAL MANAGEMENT OF CIGARETTE SMOKING

In contrast to coronary-risk factors such as high blood pressure, which may be seen as a response to a complex set of physiological triggers, cigarette smoking can be represented as a distinct and simple behavior. Evidence documenting the psychological and social conditions underlying the establishment and maintenance of this behavior is both strong and well documented (Pechacek & McAlister, 1980). The establishment of cigarette smoking, particularly in adolescents, would seem to be strongly influenced by the operation of favorable parental attitudes toward smoking and pressure from peer groups to become involved in smoking behavior. While the maintenance of smoking behavior in the adult is clearly determined by a complex mix of psychological and social conditions, the reinforcing effects of nicotine inhalation and its role in learned behavior is backed by sound evidence (Schachter, 1978). Not surprisingly, therefore, the behavioral control of smoking has proved to be a productive and copious area of research (Orleans, Shipley, Williams, & Haac, 1981).

A number of large and expensive trials based on the techniques of community education using wide media coverage have been employed both to enhance the prevention of smoking in adolescents and promote smoking cessation in adults. The results of neither have been encouraging (McAlister, Perry, & Maccoby, 1979; Thompson, 1978). While such programs have both enhanced community awareness of cigarette smoking as a risk factor for illness and produced attitude changes in favor of smoking cessation, they have failed to establish clinically useful reductions in the behavior of smoking itself (Pechacek & McAlister, 1980). This overview will not, therefore, cover community-education programs to any large extent, but instead will concentrate on smoking cessation strategies aimed at individuals or small groups, emphasizing those procedures consistent with the management of continuing risk in the cardiac patient.

The degree of attention given to studies of the behavioral control of smoking in the past decade is indicated by the work of Orleans et al. (1981) where, having scanned the relevant literature between 1969 and 1979, and sampled only those studies fulfilling certain methodological criteria, they were able to produce a bibliography containing 335 references to controlled studies of smoking cessation. These were systematically sorted into 28 topical areas of interest. Scrutiny of the number of citations appearing under each shows that most attention (though in the early rather than later parts of the decade) has been given to procedures based on aversion principles. This is followed by procedures based on self-control (self-monitoring and stimulus control), with studies of cognitive strategies, systematic desensitization, relaxation techniques, and traditional psychotherapy following behind. This breakdown provides an appropriate framework for a selective review of the evidence.

3.1   Aversion Strategies

Given the trends in behavior modification a decade or more ago (Yates, 1970), it is not surprising that aversion strategies formed a prominent focus for research into smoking cessation. The pairing of cigarette smoking behavior with an aversive stimulus, typically an electric shock or a nausea-inducing agent, has been used with mixed success in the elimination of cigarette smoking. Several systematic studies (Lichtenstein & Keutzer, 1969; Nelson, 1977; Russell, Armstrong, & Patel, 1976) have shown that aversive conditioning is of limited to moderate success in eliminating smoking behavior—at least in the short term. Moreover, others (Gerson & Lanyon, 1972) showed that the effects of aversive conditioning could be enhanced when combined with a desensitization procedure in the modification of smoking behavior.

The long-term efficacy of electric shock or nausea mediated aversion in the elimination of smoking behavior has, however, been critically questioned (Pechacek & McAlister, 1980), largely because of doubts that such aversion strategies can effectively generalize to situations outside the psychological laboratory or beyond the termination of direct treatment.

A variant on the use of physical or physiological aversion strategies is that of covert sensitization (Cautela, 1970), where the smoking behavior is paired with an imagined situation portraying aversive or unpleasant effects. Once more, however, while this procedure has been found effective in reducing smoking in the short term, there is doubt as to its durability (Bernstein & McAlister, 1976), and it is recommended more as an aid to the long-term maintenance of smoking cessation than as the primary strategy for the modification of this behavior.

The use of cigarette smoke itself as an aversive stimulus has recently attracted a good deal of interest in the research literature (Orleans et al., 1981). This has taken the form either of satiation, where numbers of cigarettes considerably in excess of an individual's normal smoking rate are consumed in a given period of time (Resnick, 1968) or rapid smoking, where the time taken to smoke each cigarette is speeded up so that the amount of inhaled cigarette smoke becomes unpleasantly high. Early studies on smoking satiation (Resnick, 1968) produced encouraging results both in the short term and long term, with around two-thirds of subjects able to eliminate or substantially curtail smoking behavior over the period of treatment. Failure to replicate this work (Claiborn, Lewis, & Humble, 1972) has, however, led to a more cautious evaluation of satiation as an effective means for the control of smoking behavior.

The literature on the rapid smoking technique (Danaher, 1977) has been both more encouraging and more consistent. Schmahl, Lichtenstein, and Harris (1972) were able to demonstrate both the short-term and long-term effectiveness of rapid smoking in the elimination of smoking among habitual smokers. The rapid smoking technique has also been shown to be superior to, or as effective as, smoking satiation (Best, Owen, & Trentadue, 1978), self-management using a specially prepared patient manual for smoking self-control (Glasgow, 1978) and both stimulus control and contractual management (Lando, 1978). Danaher (1977) also found rapid smoking to be an effective accompaniment to behavioral self-control techniques in the elimination or reduction of smoking behavior.

Evidence for the effectiveness of the rapid smoking technique has not, however, been wholly supportive, with some later studies failing to replicate the high rates of smoking cessation evident in the earlier work (Pechacek & McAlister, 1980). While this failure to replicate may be partly attributed to deviations from rapid smoking procedures used in earlier studies (Pechacek & McAlister, 1980), a suitably cautious interpretation of the data continues to be recommended.

In addition to this, the rapid smoking technique carries a particular hazard for the cardiac patient. The medical risk attached to rapid smoking, both for patients with cardiac and pulmonary diseases, is not insubstantial. This risk is associated both with the intake of excessive amounts of nicotine (with its subsequent cardiac stimulatory action) and carbon monoxide (with an associated depletion of oxygen supplies to the myocardium) (Horan, Hackett, Nicholas, Linberg, Stone, & Lukaski, 1977; Sachs & Hall, 1979). The suitability of the rapid smoking technique for the control of smoking behavior in the cardiac patient is, therefore, rather limited (Hauser, 1976), and, at the very least, this technique should be preceded by a clinical examination and the express permission of the patient's physician. Tori (1978) reported that a smoking satiation procedure involving the retention of smoke in the mouth without inhaling over a lengthy period of time was as effective as rapid smoking in the elimination of smoking behavior but did not carry the medical risks associated with the latter technique. While this may signal a potential user for smoke aversion procedures in the treatment of smoking behavior in cardiac patients, the medical risk must be fully evaluated before it becomes a treatment of prominence.

Therefore, while the technique of rapid smoking shows some promise in relatively healthy subjects, and while the combination of rapid smoking and self-control techniques offer a potentially powerful means for smoking cessation (Danaher, 1977), the single use of aversion strategies for smoking cessation would seem to be of limited use for the cardiac patient burdened with a vulnerable myocardium.

3.2   Self-Control Strategies

The major alternative to aversion strategies in the elimination or reduction of smoking behavior lies in the area of behavioral self-control. This involves an obligation on the part of the patient to remove the control of smoking behavior from situational or environmental determinants and to place it under individual control. An implicit assumption underlying most of the self-control strategies involves the development of an awareness of those stimuli in the environment which either initiate a desire for cigarettes or maintain this behavior once initiated.

Contractual management, in which the patient undertakes by way of a written contract to reduce or eliminate smoking over a period of time decided upon after consultation with a therapist (Hallaq, 1976), has produced some encouraging results in the area of smoking cessation. A number of studies have evaluated this process either singly (Lewittes & Israel, 1975; Spring, Sipich, Trimble, & Goeckner, 1978) or in combination with other techniques (Lando, 1977), and have reported smoking reduction and cessation rates in both the short- and long-terms to be appreciably in excess of those expected by placebo effects alone.

Behavioral self-monitoring, in which the patient undertakes a process involving the systematic monitoring and recording of all smoking behaviors (Israel, Raskin, & Pravder, 1979) has also been found to be a useful means toward smoking reduction and cessation. The theoretical underpinnings of behavioral self-monitoring are firmly established within the literature on behavior therapy (Rimm & Masters, 1979), and the utility of this technique both for smoking and other forms of behavioral control has been critically though favorably reviewed (Kanfer, 1970).

The technique most commonly employed in behavioral self-monitoring involves the attachment of a small record sheet to the cigarette packet such that everytime a cigarette is removed prior to smoking, a note is made of that cigarette and the circumstances surrounding its consumption, for example time of day, situation, and mood state. This technique has been successfully demonstrated in the control of smoking (both cessation and reduction) in a number of single treatment, evaluative studies (McFall, 1970; McGrath & Hall, 1976; Foxx & Brown, 1979). It has also been used as a component in comprehensive smoking-cessation programs (Hackett & Horan, 1977); and while it is difficult to dissect the effects of self-monitoring from other procedures for behavioral control employed in comprehensive packages, it has been argued that self-monitoring of smoking behavior contributes uniquely to the overall success of such programs. The empirical evidence in support of behavioral self-monitoring, together with the simplicity of the technique, make it an attractive treatment for the control of smoking behavior.

The technique of stimulus control, while somewhat more intricate than self-monitoring, also rests on the principle of subject awareness of the conditions initiating and maintaining smoking behavior. In a sense, stimulus control extends beyond self-monitoring, to the extent that the technique encourages subjects not only to record situations determining smoking behavior but also to systematically eliminate smoking behavior from those situations. This brings it under the control of more and more limited stimulus situations until the conditions under which normal rates of smoking can be undertaken become too difficult to comply with. Situational influences have been found to exert important effects on smoking behavior (Epstein & Collins, 1977), and a modest degree of evidence (Shapiro, Schwartz, Tursky, & Schnidman, 1971; Greenberg & Altman, 1976) supports the efficacy of stimulus control as an effective means of reducing or eliminating smoking behavior. Since it presents no physiological challenge to the cardiovascular system, stimulus control, either singly or in concert with other behavioral-control procedures would also, therefore, appear to offer some promise in the treatment of smoking behavior among cardiac patients.

The collective evidence on behavioral self-control strategies for the reduction or elimination of smoking is generally favorable. Recent reviews (Pechacek & McAlister, 1980), have urged some caution to the degree, firstly, that smoking cessation rates in some studies have not gone appreciably beyond expectations arising from placebo conditions and, secondly, that where smoking cessation has been achieved, it has not been a long-standing phenomenon, with recidivism arising as an important but consistent difficulty. These objections notwithstanding, the procedures of behavioral self-control are both simple to apply and do not carry with them the dangers of smoke-aversion strategies, and they must, therefore, be given some credence in the search for effective means of smoking control in the cardiac patient.

3.3   Cognitive Strategies

The role of cognitive factors in the initiation and maintenance of smoking behavior is documented by only a small literature (Steffy, Meichenbaum, & Best, 1970; Blittner, Goldberg, & Merbaum, 1978). However, several studies have evaluated the effectiveness of cognitive strategies for smoking cessation. The essence of these strategies is the development of an awareness of thought patterns or self-dialogues initiating smoking behavior and the systematic cognitive restructuring of these. The most commonly used technique has been that of thought stopping (Wisocki & Rooney, 1974; Lamontagne & Gagnon, 1978), where the thought to commence smoking has been countermanded by an imposed, opposing thought of equal strength. Results of these studies indicate that thought stopping alone can play an effective role in the reduction or cessation of smoking behavior. Moreover, there is evidence that cognitive strategies used in conjunction with smoking cessation procedures, result in at least short-term reductions in smoking behavior (Lichtenstein & Keutzer, 1969; Richards & Perri, 1978). The evidence on cognitive strategies for the control of smoking behavior remains, however, too sparse to allow definite comments about the broad utility of these techniques. In relation to the cardiac patient, it should once more be remembered that cognitive strategies pose no physiological challenge to a vulnerable myocardium.

3.4   Relaxation and Desensitization Strategies

There is only a very small body of evidence in support of the effectiveness of progressive muscle relaxation as the sole means of reduction or elimination of smoking behavior (Katz, 1979). The combination of relaxation exercises with a systematic desensitization procedure aimed at the progressive reduction of the urge to smoke in a variety of situations where smoking might normally occur, has been found to produce noticeable changes in levels of smoking behavior (Morganstern & Ratliff, 1969; Wagner & Bragg, 1970; Gerson & Lanyou, 1972). The collective evidence on the effectiveness of relaxation and systematic desensitization for the control of smoking behavior is not, however, encouraging to this point.

3.5   Physicians' Advice

Advice to stop smoking, particularly for patients with cardiac or respiratory diseases, is perhaps one of the most common exhortations made by the physician. Several attempts have been made to evaluate the effectiveness of this advice. On the surface, one might predict the success of this simple strategy to be relatively high given the potential motivation for behavior change in individuals with smoking-related illnesses. The equivocal nature of the results underscores, however, the potential strength of the smoking habit as a counterbalance to the motivation to change a behavior.

Clinical trials on the effectiveness of physicians' advice on smoking cessation have been undertaken with a diversity of groups, including those with chronic chest disease (Burns, 1969), pregnant women (Donovan, 1977), patients with myocardial infarction (Burt, Thornley, Illingsworth, White, Shaw, & Turner, 1974) and healthy individuals with one or more risk factors for coronary heart disease (Rose & Hamilton, 1978). This last study provided a representative and encouraging set of results. A random half of a large sample of middle-aged men at high risk of cardiorespiratory disease was advised by a physician of the potentially dangerous consequences of the continuation to smoke on their future health status. They were given brief but nondetailed instructions on smoking cessation, but no further intervention was undertaken. One year after this advice was given, 51% of the group had stopped smoking and has remained abstinent; most others in the group reported substantial reductions in their smoking behavior. By contrast, the group given no advice to stop smoking continued to consume cigarettes at essentially unchanged rates.

Similar results have been reported in other studies where the intervention procedure simply involved advice by a physician or other health-care worker that continuation of smoking would substantially increase the risk of future illness (Mausner, Mausner, & Rial, 1968; Meyer & Henderson, 1974; Russell, Wilson, Taylor, & Baker, 1979), and while there has been demonstrated variation between physicians in terms of the effectiveness of advice to stop smoking on smoking cessation rates (Pincherle & Wright, 1970), perhaps related to such factors as physicians' effectiveness in communication or commitment by the physician to the notion that smoking is a risk factor for cardiac or respiratory diseases, the evidence collectively seems to favor the overall usefulness of physician's advice as a means of convincing individuals to stop smoking. Physicians' advice appears to be most effective where the patient is suffering from a demonstrable set of symptoms that might be related to the inhalation of cigarette smoke and least effective where the patient is considered by the physician to be at risk of illness but where no specific symptoms can be subjectively recognized by the patient. In this respect, however, the cardiac patient would seem well suited for the use of physician or other health-care worker advice and this procedure too needs to be given careful consideration, at least as an adjunct to more active strategies, in the selection of smoking-cessation programs following heart attack.

3.6   Smoking Cessation in Cardiac Patients

As will be evident from the previous section, the results of even the most simple cessation strategy are frequently more impressive among individuals with manifest smoking-related illness than among general population samples. The bulk of this evidence comes from studies employing large samples of individuals with identified high risk of cardiac or respiratory disease (Meyer & Henderson, 1974; Rose & Hamilton, 1978). A small number of studies have, however, investigated the efficacy of smoking cessation programs in specific samples of survivors of myocardial infarction. These have typically employed only minimal intervention of the physician-advice kind, where the smoking-cessation program frequently did not extend beyond exhortations by the physician to stop smoking and very simple guidelines as to how to achieve this. Despite the simplicity of these programs, smoking-cessation rates in excess of 50% and enduring over one or more years have been reported (Burt et al., 1974; Croog & Richards, 1977; Hay & Turbott, 1970; Weinblatt et al., 1971). The chances of eliminating smoking behavior as a risk factor in the cardiac patient employing unintrusive or physiologically nonchallenging strategies would therefore appear to be encouraging.

3.7   Overview

Smoking cessation research is clearly an area with a wide diversity of strategies and an equally wide array of results. Evidence emerging from well-controlled laboratory studies employing strictly formulated behavioral strategies indicate quite reasonable success in the elimination or reduction of smoking behavior. The failure, however, of these strategies to generalize outside the laboratory and the tendency toward recidivism in even the most initially successful programs call for some caution in the interpretation of smoking-cessation research data. Moreover, the use of smoking-cessation strategies with the cardiac patient bring with them particular considerations and medical cautions that must be observed.

The effectiveness of any smoking-cessation strategy needs to be judged against the placebo effect which accompanies nonspecific interventions. This would appear to range between 15% and 25% for any control condition offered under the guise of a smoking-cessation program. While reports of smoking-cessation rates in excess of this may be found in the literature documenting the whole range of smoking-cessation strategies, there are some categories of treatments—particularly those related to cognitive restructuring, relaxation, and desensitization strategies—where the advantages in excess of the placebo effect are equivocal.

Data documenting the effectiveness of behavioral strategies for the control of smoking frequently take two forms—one to do with rates of total smoking cessation, the other to do with reductions in the frequency of cigarette consumption. Epidemiological evidence relating cigarette smoking to cardiovascular disease indicates that there is no safe level of smoking and that while cigarette smoking remains at any level, the risk of subsequent myocardial infarction is increased. This too must be a consideration in the selection of a smoking-control program following myocardial infarction. The evidence collectively favors the smoke-aversion procedures as the more effective means of smoking cessation; stimulus-control procedures appear generally to be more successful in reducing smoking rates and maintaining abstinence or reduction. On the other hand, strategies utilizing physician's advice would seem to hold considerable promise for patients with recognized and apparent physical symptomatology. Procedures based on these, perhaps enhanced with counseling and the provision of information on the noxious effects of smoking, may be the treatments of choice, at least initially, in persuading the cardiac patient to stop smoking.

This is particularly pertinent in view of the evidence on the potentially damaging cardiopulmonary effects of rapid-smoking strategies. Clearly, such strategies may carry with them unacceptable dangers when used with cardiac patients, and these dangers effectively negate the utility of smoke-aversion strategies.

One of the most troublesome issues in smoking-cessation research has to do with the long-term maintenance of short-term effects. The evidence would indicate that, with few exceptions, the whole gamut of smoking-cessation strategies is able to produce dramatic short-term gains both in smoking cessation and reduction (Pechacek & McAlister, 1980). Moreover, while the virtues of specific smoking-cessation programs have long been debated, there is little reason to believe that any one is superior to any other (Levenberg & Wagner, 1976). However, while the immediate effects of smoking-cessation strategies give great encouragement, the long-term effects can be viewed with some disappointment. An overview of research indicates that smoking cessation rates of between 60% and 70% evident at termination of smoking-cessation programs reduce to between 20% and 30% within three months of the end of program (McFall, 1978). While this rate of recidivism has been viewed as an artifact resulting from evaluations of single therapeutic interventions with populations of self-selected subjects actively seeking help (Schachter, 1982), it nonetheless foreshadows a serious threat to the overall utility of smoking-cessation strategies and constitutes a pressing research problem in the area of the behavioral control of smoking (Pechacek & McAlister, 1980). A variety of means have been suggested to counteract this difficulty, including the use of composite programs involving specific maintenance strategies such as the continued practice of self-monitoring, the provision of assistance with the potential side effects of smoking cessation (weight gain, emotional agitation, and the like), and the incorporation into smoking-cessation programs of specific periods of follow-up that allow patient contact with the clinic and enhance the practice and effectiveness of maintenance strategies. Given the potential problems of recidivism, due attention to the issues of the maintenance of behavior change cannot be overestimated; however, this is an issue that is equally pertinent to the use of behavioral strategies for the control of other cardiac-risk factors.

Very little research has been done to evaluate the relative effectiveness of group versus individual treatment, though this issue too is common to the behavioral control of other cardiac risks and may ultimately reduce to a decision of clinical convenience.

Given the overall demand for multifocus intervention following myocardial infarction, the amount of time available for smoking cessation or other coronary risk control programs may be limited. Simple techniques involving a combination of physician advice and education, the teaching of simple monitoring procedures as a maintenance strategy, and assistance with the potential side effects of smoking cessation may, together with the motivating effects for behavior change of cardiac disease itself, add up to the most effective package for the control of smoking in the cardiac patient.

CHAPTER 7

Type A Behavior and Its Management in the Cardiac Patient

1. THE CONCEPT OF TYPE A BEHAVIOR

The contribution of Type A behavior to the risk of coronary heart disease is considered in the first chapter; it is sufficient for present purposes simply to reiterate the importance of this association. The evidence documenting it is abundant and reference to any one of a number of well-conducted epidemiological studies (for example, Rosenman et al., 1975; Haynes, Feinleib, & Kannell, 1980; Kornitzer et al., 1981) or to any of several recent critical reviews of the literature (for example, Brand, 1978; Zyzanski, 1978; Rosenman & Chesney, 1980) should serve to illustrate this point quite adequately. The evidence arising from the Western Collaborative Group Study is particularly useful in this respect, because the careful measurement of Type A behavior and its prospective association with coronary heart disease formed a distinct focus of the study. Data arising from that work showed that persons exhibiting Type A behavior suffered an 8.5-year relative risk of myocardial infarction—around twice that of persons for whom Type A behavior was absent—and that this risk was independent of the presence of other risk factors such as serum cholesterol, hypertension, and cigarette smoking (Rosenman et al., 1975). Contemporary studies on a roughly similar scale and with almost identical results—for example, the Belgian Heart Study (Kornitzer et al., 1981) or the later stages of the Framingham Study (Haynes et al., 1980)—give unarguable credibility to the use of Type A behavior as an explanatory concept in the onset of coronary heart disease.

1.1 Definitions of Type A Behavior

Definitions of Type A behavior are both broad and variable. An operational definition, which is so necessary to guide the development of intervention strategies, must really be built up from first principles. A number of existing definitions and descriptions do, however, set a useful context within which to discuss the overall notion of Type A behavior.

While the introduction of both the term and the idea of Type A behavior are undeniably attributed to the pioneering work of Friedman and Rosenman (1959, 1974), the essence of this idea was eloquently stated in the last century by Sir William Osler. In his textbook *The Principles and Practice of Medicine* Osler said of the patient with myocardial infarction that he was:

> . . . not the delicate neurotic person . . . but the robust, the vigorous in mind and body, the keen and ambitious man, the indicator of whose engines was also at full speed. (Osler, 1892.)

While this cannot be considered a definition of Type A behavior as such, it nicely portrays the attributes of ambition and time pressure that have come to be so characteristic of this behavior pattern.

Contemporary definitions are best represented by that of Friedman (1969) who defined Type A behavior as:

> A characteristic action-emotion complex which is exhibited by those individuals who are engaged in a relatively chronic struggle to obtain an unlimited number of poorly defined things from their environment in the shortest period of time, and if necessary against the opposing efforts of other persons or things in the same environment.

Glass (1977), with a rather more succinct turn of phrase, defined Type A behavior as: "A style of overt response to certain forms of stressful situations." The value of this definition and the reason that it deserves mention is not that it advances our understanding of Type A behavior as a manifest phenomenon. That role must be taken either by definitions such as that of Friedman (1969) or by descriptions of the observable or measurable elements of Type A behavior. Glass's (1977) definition does, however, tie the appearance of Type A behavior to the preceding existence of a set of environmental circumstances and establishes the behavior, *inter alia,* as a contingent if complex response to situational or environmental challenges. The experimental work upon which Glass (1977) based this definition identified those situational challenges as events over which the individual perceived little or no personal control. The concept of locus of control and response to environmental challenges (Byrne, 1980), and the concomitant state of learned helplessness (Seligman, 1975) is well known in behavioral medicine. Whether or not this builds too great a degree of specificity into the conceptualization of Type A behavior is still open to debate (Glass, 1977). However, it does bring with it the benefit of a great deal of experimental support.

A number of descriptions of Type A behavior may serve to extend these definitions into recognizable aspects of human activity. Byrne (1981) said of this phenomenon:

> The literature collectively suggests that persons manifesting this behavior pattern are characterised by a sense of time urgency, are ambitious with a high need for

achievement, are impatient and intolerant of frustration and exhibit an unusual degree of job involvement.

Herman, Blumenthal, Black, and Chesney (1981) with encouraging similarity describe the Type A individual as: ". . . typically aggressive, competitive, ambitious and hostile, with a pervasive quality of time urgency and impatience." There are of course many such descriptions. Each paper on Type A behavior seems to contain its own. However, the differences between these are subtle at most, and one can assume a fair amount of agreement as to the various components of behavior that have been observed to make up the overall pattern.

Factorial descriptions of Type A behavior tend to confirm those based on observation. Zyzanski and Jenkins (1970) use data from the Western Collaborative Group Study to examine the factor structure of responses to the Jenkins Activity Survey (Jenkins et al., 1967). This was a self-completed questionnaire designed specifically for use in the study as one of several methods for assessing the Type A Behavior Pattern. A factor analysis of these data that can be described as statistically meticulous yielded three independent factors. The first of these was termed *Hard Driving and Competitiveness*. Items significantly loading on this factor identified a pattern of behavior concerned with task commitment, expenditure of effort, and the perception of activities and interactions as challenges to be accepted and dominated. While such behaviors might be most prominently observed within the work situation, there are many other environments such as those involved in competitive sport or other activities that might allow this pattern to become manifest. The second factor was labeled *Job Involvement*. Items significantly loading on this factor were identified specifically with the work place and describe behaviors to do with the acceptance or establishment of difficult and challenging deadlines, the tendency to extend work past normal hours, the acceptance and, indeed, soliciting of work in excess of personal capacity, and the conviction that job demands should take precedence over all other considerations. The final factor attracted the label *Speed and Impatience*. This was identified by items portraying undue haste and rapidity in both motor and cognitive activities, a self-imposed time pressure, an intolerance of slowness in others, and an inordinate degree of irritability and distractability.

Reference to this study serves several purposes. Firstly, it provides empirical confirmation of the more impressionistic descriptions arising from earlier work. Secondly, it begins the process of delineating the several elements of the Type A Behavior Pattern, so establishing it as a complex and nonunitary set of behaviors. The idea that the Type A Behavior Pattern is in fact composed of a number of independent elements has recently been discussed by Jenkins and Zyzanski (1982a). Finally, the statistical work arising from this study lays the grounds for a more detailed measurement of Type A behavior, and so for the establishment of more specific associations between Type A behavior and clinically manifest cardiovascular disease.

Of course, it can always be said that factor analytic descriptions of data represent no more than the organized output of a more heterogeneous input. This argument can never be lightly discounted, though the sample size and the nature of the measuring instrument in this case guarantee reliable observations, and the identifiable character of the emerging factors gives one confidence that these factors reflect systematic rather than random responses to proffered items. Moreover, the finding of Matthews et al. (1977), that a factor analysis of another measure of Type A behavior, the Structured Interview, produced factors resembling those arising from the work of Zyzanski and Jenkins (1970), may be taken as a useful confirmation both of the earlier factorial description of Type A behavior and of the notion that it is made up of several components.

One facet of Type A behavior understated in earlier studies but recently assuming prominence is that of hostility. While the attribute of aggression appears in most descriptions of Type A behavior, its emergence either as a predictor of myocardial infarction or as an element in factorial descriptions of the behavior pattern is only now attracting interest. Both Francis (1981) and Smith (1984) have reported modest but consistent correlations between measures of Type A behavior and self-reported expressions of anger and hostility. In addition, more recent factorial examinations of common methods of assessing the Type A Behavior Pattern have indicated hostility to be a notable component of the pattern (Anderson & Waldron, 1983; Matthews et al., 1982). Prospective studies (Barefoot, Dahlstrom, & Williams, 1983; Shekelle, Gayle, Ostfeld, & Paul, 1983; Williams, Haney, Lee, Kong, Blumenthal, & Whalen, 1980) have significantly related both to risk of coronary heart disease and mortality from it. Moreover, a more modest study of the experience of angina in patients with diagnosed coronary artery disease (Smith, Follick, & Korr, 1984) showed that the frequency of angina attacks was quite strongly related to the possession of self-reported anger. Data such as these would indicate that future work on the relationship between Type A behavior and coronary heart disease should not ignore the potentially important role of anger and hostility as components of the former.

1.2   The Origins of Type A Behavior

There has been remarkably little research as to how the Type A Behavior Pattern arises, though this is an aspect of the subject that has been clearly identified as a research priority (Dembroski, Weiss, Shields, Haynes, & Feinleib, 1978) in view of its bearing on intervention (Gentry & Suinn, 1978).

There is little evidence that Type A behavior has a genetic basis. Studies of Type A behavior in both monozygotic and dyzygotic twins (Rosenman, Rahe, Borhani, & Feinleib, 1976) and on similarities in Type A behavior between twins and their parents (Matthews & Krantz, 1976) gave no support to an argument that

Type A behavior can be transmitted by means of the gene complement. A reanalysis of the Rosenman data (Matthews et al., 1984) did, however, reveal a possible genetic influence on the potential for hostility, together with loudness of speech and competition for control of the interview during a structured interview assessment of the Type A Behavior Pattern. The strength of the genetic argument appears to some extent dependent on the way in which Type A behavior is measured (Cohen, Matthews, & Waldron, 1978), though hypotheses regarding the heritability of Type A behavior are not at present given broad credibility.

Social and cultural factors are somewhat more likely progenitors of Type A behavior—though, once more, the evidence is not strong and rather more circumstantial than direct. Sex differences in Type A behavior have been demonstrated (Waldron, Zyzanski, Shekelle, Jenkins, & Tannenbaum, 1977), with men more strongly exhibiting the behavior pattern than women. While this may be interpreted to represent a differential effect of socialization, it might show nothing more than that the procedures used to measure Type A behavior are biassed in favour of male responses.

Quite prominent crosscultural differences in Type A behavior are also evident (Cohen, 1978). By and large these differences are consistent with expectations, in the sense that Type A behavior is most commonly seen in those cultures where competition and achievement are valued. This point is suitably illustrated by Cohen, Syme, Jenkins, Kagan and Zyzanski (1975), in reporting data on Type A behavior among Japanese in traditional and nontraditional cultures. Even so, Cohen (1978) cautioned that data of these kinds are too ambiguous to allow confident inferences on cultural determinants of Type A behavior. One might assume this to be particularly so since the instruments designed to measure Type A behavior in one cultural context may not be readily transportable to another.

Both Chesney, Eagleston, and Rosenman, (1981) and Mettlin (1976) have taken up the point that Westernized urban societies, particularly those parts of them which have to do with commerce and professional activity, actually make it difficult for a person to succeed without manifesting at least some components of the Type A Behavior Pattern. While this may be more pertinent to the maintenance of Type A behavior than to its origins, it should be borne in mind that even the most logical attempts at the modification of Type A behavior may be forced to do battle with the conflicting demands of well-established social and cultural demands.

Perhaps the most promising evidence on the origins of Type A behavior comes from developmental studies. Matthews (1978), in reviewing the small literature on the developmental antecedents of Type A behavior, concluded that: "There is converging evidence that parental standards of performance, which are ever escalating, play a role in the etiology of Type A behavior . . ." Therefore, just as it is inherently sensible that prevailing social demands and attitudes might initiate and reinforce Type A behaviors in the adult, it is equally sensible that observed parental attitudes and demands might establish this pattern of behavior in children. There is now evidence that practices of child rearing play an important role in the development of Type A behavior (Matthews & Glass, 1977; Matthews, 1978), particularly for the attributes of achievement motivation and aggression (Matthews, 1978). There is little evidence to implicate developmental influences on time urgency.

Data on the origins of Type A behavior are, therefore, somewhat sparse and fragmented, but a coherent picture is beginning to emerge. The most likely source of the behavior pattern is to be found within the developmental experiences to which the individual is exposed during childhood. Thus, while a prevailing social climate might provide the conditions under which Type A behaviors can become manifest and might also reward those behaviors when they emerge, the initial tendency to respond with Type A behaviors to appropriate environmental challenges would seem to have been laid down during childhood.

1.3   Emotion and Type A Behavior

The relationship between Type A behavior and emotion or affect is contentious. By tradition, the overt experience of emotional distress among those exhibiting Type A behavior has been denied. Jenkins (1978) quite explicitly stated:

> The developers of the Type A concept have emphasized that the behavior pattern is not a reflection of stress, anxiety, or psychological disturbance . . . neither the interview nor the JAS [both measures of Type A behavior] have been found to correlate significantly with a wide variety of measures of emotional distress or psychological dysfunction.

This contrasts, to an extent, with Friedman's (1969) conception of Type A behavior which, *inter alia,* refers to ". . . an action-emotion complex . . ." and conveys the impression that both activity and affect are interrelated manifestations of the Type A response. More recent evidence, too, would seem to challenge the unequivocal acceptance of the statement that Type A behavior and emotion are entirely unrelated. Byrne (1981) showed that Type A behavior scores among cardiac patients correlated with the tendency to attribute undue affective distress to encountered life events. While one might argue that such results may be contaminated by the fact that patients were interviewed during the time immediately following their myocardial infarction, the result has been confirmed in samples of healthy subjects (Byrne & Rosenman, 1985). The work of Dimsdale, Hackett, Block, and Hutter (1978), which showed modest but significant correlations between measures of Type A behavior and measures of accumulated stressful life events, together with present state measures of tension, depressive mood, and anger, supports this position.

More recently, reports have appeared in the literature to document associations between measures of Type A behavior and a range of indices both of neurosis and of symptoms of affective distress. The most extreme representation of this has been the claim, based on correlations between measures of Type A behavior and neuroticism, that the two bear sufficiently close conceptual similarities that the former might be considered a category of the latter (Eysenck & Fulker, 1982; Irvine, Lyle, & Allon, 1982; Bass, 1984). Studies focussing on the state nature of emotional discomfort have, however, provided the bulk of the evidence.

Bass (1984) reported a strong association between self-reported Type A behavior and a measure of conspicuous psychiatric symptomatology in a sample of men with chest pain. Smith (1984) presented evidence of significant correlations between self-reported Type A behavior and both state anger and neuroticism, again in a sample of patients with identified angina.

Lest the use of patient samples be seen as too prone to potential contamination, supportive data have also emerged from studies of subjects without manifest coronary disease. Francis (1981) reported that Type A students facing the challenge of examinations were more likely than their Type B colleagues to experience anxiety, depression, and hostility, while Chesney et al. (1981), in a large study of healthy adult males, revealed small but significant correlations between self-report (but not interview) measures of Type A behavior and a variety of self-assessed indices of both state and trait anxiety and of depression. Though this latter study takes the view that emergent correlations reflect, as much as anything, the failure of self-report measures of the Type A Behavior Pattern to adequately assess the construct, the fact remains that scales of Type A behavior shown to predict coronary heart disease also correlate clearly with measures of emotional discomfort. Data reported by Wadden, Anderson, Foster, and Love (1983) indicate more selective associations, with self-report measures of Type A behavior relating significantly to state and trait anxiety but not to standard indices of underlying psychiatric impairment.

The role of emotion in Type A behavior is important in any consideration of the modification of this behavior pattern, as intervention strategies are likely to be aimed not only at the overt behaviors but also at the consequences of these behaviors.

1.4 Psychophysiological Correlates of Type A Behavior

Data from studies of both autonomic and neuroendocrinological functioning among Type A persons indicates that, at least during periods of manifest Type A behavior, the individual may be characterized by levels of elevated sympathetic arousal (Steptoe, 1981). Jennings and Choi (1981) examined several parameters of cardiovascular activation among Type A subjects during the execution of cognitive tasks requiring motor responses. Physiological responsivity of Type A subjects was seen to vary with degree of task demand. Dembroski and colleagues

(1977, 1978) reported significant increases in both heart rate and blood pressure among Type A subjects relative to their non–Type A counterparts when presented with challenging cognitive tasks. Similar results with regard to increases in blood pressure were reported by Manuck and Garland (1979), though Pittner and Houston (1980) suggested that blood pressure responses of this kind in Type A subjects were, at least in part, a function of the nature of the stressor.

Results in this area have not, however, been wholly positive. Scherwitz, Berton, & Leventhal (1978) found no association between Type A behavior and cardiovascular reactivity during a variety of tasks designed to elicit the Type A response. Moreover, neither Lundberg and Forsman (1979) nor Frankenhaeuser, Lundberg, and Forsman (1980a) were able to show heart rate effects among Type A subjects under a range of conditions of cognitive challenge representing both under- and overstimulation. Steptoe (1981) and Steptoe and Ross (1981) suggested that these results may be attributed to the use of discontinuous measures of cardiovascular activation. They therefore employed continuous measures both of blood pressure and of heart-rate parameters to determine whether this improvement in methodology produced more consistent associations between cardiovascular reactivity and Type A behavior. Once more, the results were unable to demonstrate unequivocal associations. Whether this seriously weakens the pathophysiological argument linking Type A behavior with coronary-artery pathology is debatable, though Steptoe and Ross (1981) quite firmly imply that an association of some kind must exist.

A parallel line of research has involved the use of measures of adrenocortical functioning as an index of sympathetic arousal. Frankenhaeuser et al. (1980b) demonstrated significantly higher rises in urinary catecholamine output among Type A subjects who were forcibly kept inactive than among non–Type A subjects who were subjected to the same conditions. This relates to the notion that understimulation and inactivity are particularly aversive to those endowed with Type A attributes. Lundberg and Forsman (1979) showed similarly that excretion of cortisol was significantly higher among Type A subjects than among non–Type A subjects during conditions of sensory understimulation, while significant differences in the same direction emerged for catecholamine excretion during conditions of overstimulation. Differences between sympathetic-adrenal and pituitary-adrenal output for Type A and non–Type A subjects under conditions of self-paced achievement were not evidenced in the results of Frankenhaeuser et al. (1980a), though the task conditions varied considerably from those of Lundberg and Forsman (1979), and it is possible that the characteristics of the situational demand or challenge have a determining effect on the psychophysiological response (Glass, 1978; Pittner & Houston, 1980).

More recently, a number of studies have adopted a somewhat different perspective, in that rather than postulating a relationship between aspects of the situational challenge and measures of psychophysiological arousal, they have suggested distinctive associations between components of the Type A Behavior Pattern itself and potential for psychophysiological arousal. In these studies, the component of time urgency or speed and impatience has emerged as the predominant precipitant of cardiovascular activation.

Jennings (1984) showed that impatient and competitive behavior could be elicited by a choice reaction-time task involving low monetary reward, and that during task trials (but not between them), subjects with these attributes of Type A behavior showed a brief, intense cardiovascular involvement with sympatheticlike physiological changes. Heart-rate changes were also evident in young boys (average age, 10 years) identified as impatient and aggressive by a children's test of Type A behavior, when they were challenged with a cognitive/motor task requiring anticipation and accurate responding (Jennings & Matthews, 1984). Using a different measure of biological activation, Madsen and McGuire (1984) found a number of measures of Type A behavior, and particularly those to do with speed and impatience, to be significantly related to whole blood serotonin (5-hydroxytryptamine). While this evidence must necessarily be seen as tentative, it raises the possibility that some components of the Type A Behavior Pattern may, in the long term, prove more cardiotoxic than others.

The evidence relating Type A behavior to psychophysiological dysfunction or to patterns of hemodynamic disturbance is, on the whole, somewhat variable. A major review considering the findings of 45 studies examining the psychophysiological concomitants of Type A behavior (Myrtek & Greenlee, 1984) was unable to find any consistent pattern of physiological activation among Type A subjects presented with a range of challenge situations which distinguished them reliably from Type B subjects. The bulk of this evidence, however, supports the argument that Type A individuals will, under some circumstances, respond to environmental challenges with potentially damaging physiological responses. There is, of course, a rather longer step between such evidence as this and the establishment of specific pathological links between Type A behavior and coronary-artery pathology. Some evidence would indicate that the presence of elevated levels of catecholamines in the blood facilitates the production of endogenous cholesterol (Friedman & Rosenman, 1974) and it is reasonably widely accepted that under similar conditions, platelets are more likely to aggregate together in the production of arterial thrombosis (Ardlie, Glew & Schwartz, 1966). Research on these aspects of Type A behavior is, however, a very clear priority and is likely to become a substantial focus of work in the near future.

1.5   Overview

The material presented in the preceding sections may be seen as representative of a growing body of empirical evidence which both links the presence of Type A behavior to the onset of cardiovascular disease and describes the nature and consequences of Type A behavior. The literature on Type A behavior has, of course, been well reviewed in other publications (Rosenman & Chesney, 1981;

Chesney et al., 1981) and any of these will serve to further familiarize the reader with the diverse range of investigations pertinent to this topic. The clinical task of designing effective intervention strategies for individuals with Type A behavior, either as a preventive or treatment exercise, could be best addressed if this large body of literature could be integrated into some cohesive model that delineates the various components of Type A behavior and the several consequences of these. Such a theoretical model need not necessarily represent the intricate details of what is surely a complex set of processes. Though, in view of the stance that behavioral medicine advocates a systematic rather than intuitive approach to intervention, a model of this kind should be seen as a necessary conceptual step.

Though the origins of Type A behavior are not yet adequately understood, the evidence points most strongly to the idea that through developmental experiences, and particularly those in which the child interacts with its parents, a set of attitudes or cognitive interpretations of the social environment are acquired that will ultimately determine the ways in which the adult will respond to that environment. This should not be taken to imply the development of an enduring personality trait. It simply indicates that at some stage during the child's developmental experiences, patterns of behavioral organization or cognitive sets will be laid down which, in adult life, will interact with situational challenges or demands made by the social environment to produce manifest responses identifiable as Type A behaviors. In this sense, it is not unlike the formulations of personality put forward by Mischel (1976), where the situational determinants of "personality" are given considerable prominence. The first stage of a model linking the various aspects of Type A behavior might thus be seen as a developmental stage that results in patterns of organizational set and leads, eventually, to the determination of behavioral responses to environmental demands.

A useful parallel to this conceptualization lies in the work of Lazarus (1966), where the organismic response of stress is seen to arise, not so much as a function of the nature of the environment, as the result of cognitive strategies laid down during development, which provide an interpretive filter for individual experiences. The value of including such a phase in any conceptual model of Type A behavior and its consequences, particularly where this model is directed toward intervention, is that such postulated cognitive filters would seem to be amenable to restructuring (Meichenbaum, 1977). The first line of intervention may, therefore, be to attempt to restructure those cognitive interpretations which translate environmental experiences into manifest episodes of Type A behavior.

The next stage in the model has to do with the overt behaviors that result from the interaction between the individual and his or her environment. The characteristic nature of these behaviors is described earlier in this chapter. Friedman and Rosenman (1974) provide a useful list of specific behaviors which are readily identifiable, both to the health professional and to the lay person. Clearly, such overt behaviors will vary from one person to another and, indeed, from one situation to another. Specific behaviors which, for example, may be observed in the home situation, might be qualitatively and thematically different from those which are produced in the work place (Chesney & Rosenman, 1980; Thoresen & Öhman, 1985). Indeed, there has never been a suggestion in the literature on Type A behavior that all persons who exhibit this behavior pattern will be characterized by each and every component or aspect of it, or that situations that produce the Type A response will be consistent from one person to another. As with any clinical phenomenon, interindividual variability is both expected and important. In this respect, while intervention at the behavioral level is perhaps the most clear-cut of all, it is crucial that the nature of such behaviors in any individual is both identified and described prior to the implementation of intervention.

The consequences of Type A behaviors form the final stage of this model and take several forms. While some (Jenkins, 1978) hold that Type A persons neither experience nor report distress, and others present evidence that the effective use of denial and repression among Type A persons may mask subjective distress (Vickers, Hervig, Rahe, & Rosenman, 1981), there is increasing doubt that distress is a phenomenon totally absent from the Type A pattern (Byrne, 1981). Indeed, Suinn (1980) suggests that the management of distress is an essential element in the modification of Type A behavior. Its potential existence must, therefore, be recognized and included into any systematic organization of components in this area.

Psychophysiological consequences, too, would appear to be important, at least when persons are behaving in Type A ways. At this level, a state of sympathetic hyperarousal, largely evident within the cardiovascular system, presents as a focus for intervention (Surwit et al., 1981).

Finally, one must consider the social, personal, and occupational consequences of Type A behavior, for within particular social settings, these may be powerful reinforcers of the behavior pattern. It might be suggested that the gains arising from Type A behavior are rather more illusory than actual, and the belief among Type A persons that speed and impatience and job involvement equate, for example, with superior efficiency is not borne out by the evidence. Intervention at this level may best be seen as relying on information giving and reassurance, together with a re-evaluation of social demands and the possible advantages and disadvantages that these may bring about.

Each of these foci of intervention will be discussed in rather more detail when specific studies of and approaches to intervention are considered later in this chapter.

2. MEASUREMENT OF TYPE A BEHAVIOR

The measurement of Type A behavior assumes several important roles within the context of intervention. Firstly, the presence and extent of Type A behavior needs to be established in some systematic way. Secondly, if the object of the exercise is to modify this behavior, then the effectiveness of that modification strategy needs to be evaluated, and this involves systematic measurement both before and after the application of any intervention strategy. Finally, since Type A behavior is not a unitary concept but is made up of several distinct elements (Zyzanski & Jenkins, 1970; Jenkins & Zyzanski, 1982) and since these elements are neither uniformly related to the risk of coronary heart disease (Jenkins, 1978) nor evenly distributed among all those exhibiting Type A behavior (Chesney, Eagleston & Rosenman, 1981), it would seem useful to know, for any single individual, the relative presence of the components of Type A behavior so that appropriate foci for intervention could be adopted.

Innes and Clark (1980) reported at least seven verbal measures of the Type A Behavior Pattern in current use. Of course not all of these measures are uniformly related to the risk of coronary heart disease (Rosenman, 1978); this reflects the diversity of attitudes, behaviors, and feelings which have been observed to make up the total constellation of Type A behaviors. Useful reviews of this field may be obtained from several sources (Byrne, Rosenman, Schiller, & Chesney, 1985; Chesney et al., 1981) and the psychometric properties of the various Type A measuring instruments has been particularly well covered by Caffrey (1978).

Two measures of Type A behavior are most commonly used. These are the structured interview (Rosenman, Friedman, & Straus, 1975; Rosenman, 1978) and the Jenkins Activity Survey (Jenkins, Zyzanski, & Rosenman, 1979). Considerable debate exists as to the relative efficacy of these two.

2.1   The Structured Interview

This was first developed for use in the Western Collaborative Group Study and reports of associations between Type A behavior and myocardial infarction have arisen largely from its use (Rosenman et al., 1975). In view of strong and consistent associations between categorizations of Type A behavior based on the Structured Interview and the onset of various manifestations of cardiovascular disease, this technique has achieved a useful reputation as a Type A measure. The qualitative and thematic structure of the interview arose from a series of clinical observations that were cast in the form of questions or other forms of information-gathering interactions. These set out to address (a) the degree of drive and ambition, (b) the degree of past and present aggressive competitive hostile feelings, and (c) the degree of time urgency (Chesney et al., 1981) exhibited by an individual. The items making up the Structured Interview are presented in detail by these authors. These items are administered as part of an interview in such a way that the interviewer is not only able to note the verbal content of subjects' responses but is also able to establish "a Type A environment" for the interview. Thus, the person with Type A predispositions is actually encouraged to display these in response to challenges during the interview.

This is achieved, for example, by the interviewer omitting to complete the ends of sentences, so that the Type A person, in order to rush through, will go on ahead of the interviewer. The interviewer is, therefore, able to note actual instances of Type A behavior when they occur throughout the interview.

On the basis both of verbal responses to questions and of judgments of actual instances of Type A behavior manifested throughout the interview, the interviewer makes ratings concerning the presence of Type A behavior or its absence (Type B behavior), and also of the degree to which Type A or Type B behaviors are apparent. A five-point scale is used to give the following distinctions:

A1: Fully developed Type A pattern;
A2: Many Type A characteristics, but not the complete pattern;
 X: An even mix of Type A and Type B characteristics;
B3: Many Type B characteristics, but some Type A characteristics as well;
B4: A relative absence of Type A characteristics.

Because the Structured Interview acts as a situational challenge for Type A behaviors, the conditions surrounding the interview are crucially important. Chesney et al. (1981) point out that each interviewer must be consistent with respect to vocal style (speed, volume, intonation, and inflection), length of the interview, question content, and interviewer behavior. They describe the emotional tone of the interview as "coldly professional" and emphasize the importance that the interviewer's behavior should not vary from one subject to another. It should go without saying that where more than one interviewer is used, these criteria must not vary between interviewers.

Reliability between several interviewers has in fact been found quite acceptable. Caffrey (1968) reported inter-rater reliability coefficients as varying between 0.64 and 0.84, with the more modest correlations occurring for relatively newly trained interviewers. Test retest reliability, too, has been examined (Jenkins et al., 1968), with reliability coefficients of around 0.82 over periods of between 12 and 20 months being evident. However, in an assessment procedure where the outcome relies substantially on the subjective judgments of individuals, as opposed to the self-reported feelings and behaviors of subjects themselves, one must note carefully the possibility that collected data may become contaminated by subjective impressions. This places the Structured Interview at somewhat of a disadvantage with respect to other instruments. The other disadvantage attaching to this procedure concerns both the amount of time required to administer it and the degree of training necessary for an interviewer to become competent in its administration. Thus, while the epidemiological associations between Structured Interview established Type A behavior and coronary heart disease are persuasively high, the practical concerns to do with its administration within the clinical setting may disallow its routine use in clinical settings where self-report instruments provide a more convenient means of assessment.

2.2   The Jenkins Activity Survey

The Jenkins Activity Survey (Jenkins et al., 1979) is the major rival to the
Structured Interview in the measurement of Type A behavior. This is a self-
completed questionnaire, the content of which arose from the item content of the
interview instrument. The present version (there have been several developments
over the past years) contains 52 items (Jenkins et al., 1979). Factor analytic work
on earlier versions of this scale (Zyzanski & Jenkins, 1970) revealed the three
dimensions of hard driving and competitiveness, job involvement, speed, and
impatience. Use of the Jenkins Activity Survey produces a global Type A score
and three subscores representing the three factors just listed. The value of this
lies with the finer dissection of the substructure of the Type A Behavior Pattern.

Jenkins et al. (1979) reported a range of studies quoting rates of agreement
ranging between 71% and 73% for Jenkins Activity Survey scores with classifications of Type A behavior based on the Structured Interview. Moreover,
Chesney et al. (1981) suggested that scores on the Jenkins Activity Survey are
able to distinguish retrospectively between patients with myocardial infarction
and healthy control subjects. Zyzanski, Jenkins, Ryan, Flessas, and Everist
(1976) also reported an association between Jenkins Activity Survey scores and
degree of coronary atherosclerosis among patients who had undergone coronary
angiography. Internal reliability for the four Jenkins Activity Survey scales (the
Global Scale and three subscales) ranges between 0.73 and 0.85, while test retest
reliability over a four- to six-month interval ranges between 0.65 and 0.82
(Jenkins et al., 1979).

Chesney et al. (1981) questioned the advantages of the Jenkins Activity
Survey over the Structured Interview in at least three respects. Firstly, the prospective evidence linking Type A behavior with myocardial infarction is weaker
for Jenkins Activity Survey scores than for Structured Interview classifications
(Brand, Rosenman, Jenkins, Sholtz, & Zyzanski, 1981). Secondly, the relation
between Jenkins Activity Survey scores and coronary angiographic findings has
not been replicated (Blumenthal, Williams, Kong, Schanberg, & Thompson,
1978). Finally, Structured Interview ratings were more strongly related to cardiovascular reactivity during experimentally induced stress than were Jenkins
Activity Survey scores (Dembroski, MacDougall, Shields, Petitto, & Lushene,
1978). The Jenkins Activity Survey does, however, have the advantages both of
convenience (it is self-completed) and of dividing up the Type A Behavior
Pattern into its relative components. Thus, while the epidemiological considerations to do with strengths of association between measures of Type A behavior and incidence of coronary heart disease are of course important, the clinical utility of a self-completed instrument such as the Jenkins Activity Survey
may override these considerations within the context of clinical behavioral medicine.

2.3   Other Measures of Type A Behavior

Vickers (1973) developed a brief nine-item self-completed questionnaire for use in epidemiological surveys. This scale was found to correlate around 0.80 with the Jenkins Activity Survey and to be associated with the presence of a number of coronary-risk factors. It did not, however, distinguish between patients with myocardial infarction and those with less serious illnesses (Byrne, 1981), and has been criticized for failing to assess the entire universe of Type A behaviors (Caffrey, 1978). Therefore, while this short instrument has the advantage of being convenient and simple to use, it is unlikely to provide an adequate measure of a complex behavior pattern and cannot, therefore, be recommended for use in the clinical setting.

A scale that is almost as brief was reported by Bortner (1969), though this instrument failed to correlate at all with Jenkins Activity Survey scores. It provided a 66% agreement with classifications of Type A behavior arising from the Structured Interview, and patients with myocardial infarction were found to have higher scores on the Bortner scale than healthy control subjects (Heller, 1979). There is, however, little epidemiological evidence to link scores on this scale to prospective risk for myocardial infarction; once more, its use within the clinical context seems very limited.

Rather more epidemiological evidence has accumulated from the Framingham Study (Haynes et al., 1980), where in its latest stages, a short, self-completed instrument was developed for the assessment of Type A behavior. Items contained in this instrument were chosen on the grounds that they were "typical of the Type A Behavior Pattern." This scale was found to be a significant predictor of myocardial infarction at eight-year follow-up. The evidence linking this measure of Type A behavior with risk of myocardial infarction is rather stronger than that attached to the two previously discussed, short measures of the Type A Behavior Pattern. This immediately makes it a potential prospect as clinical measure of Type A behavior. More work is still to be done, however, on its use within the clinical context; as yet, it is unlikely to supplant the more established means for assessing Type A behavior.

Both Chesney et al. (1981) and Jenkins and Zyzanski (1982b) have reported modest correlations between standard measures of Type A behavior and scales arising from established, psychometric measures of personality. These have included the California Psychological Inventory, the activity scale of the Thurstone Temperament Schedule, and the dominance scale of the Adjective Checklist. This last scale has been examined in rather more detail in relation to Type A behavior by Herman et al. (1982). There is no evidence, however, either clinical or epidemiological, that scores on these scales relate to risk of myocardial infarction. Therefore they do not present useful alternatives for the clinical assessment of Type A behavior.

2.4   Overview

On balance there would seem to be no real challenge to the primacy of either the Structured Interview or the Jenkins Activity Survey as measures of Type A behavior. The choice between these may reduce ultimately to ease of administration and distinction between the various subtypes of Type A behavior as against the stronger epidemiological associations established between Type A behavior and coronary heart disease. The Structured Interview certainly does have the benefit of extensive epidemiological use and its psychometric properties have been well investigated and are acceptable. The clinical demands of assessment prior to intervention among persons with Type A behavior do, however, seem to point to some self-completed instrument as a more appropriate measure. Firstly, administration does not require extensive training and the expenditure of interviewer time, and these considerations are clearly important within the context of a clinical practice. Secondly, one such instrument (the Jenkins Activity Survey) identifies and separately quantifies some of the several components aking up the overall Type A Behavior Pattern. In terms of the selection of appropriate intervention strategies, this more precise assessment procedure is entirely consistent with a fundamental aim of behavior therapy—that is, to match the characteristics of the treatment to the specific problems exhibited by the patient (Yates, 1975). Moreover, this has been marked as a necessary prelude to the modification of Type A behavior (Chesney et al. 1981).

3.   THE MODIFICATION OF TYPE A BEHAVIOR

In an area where the epidemiological association between a behavior pattern and a disease category is so persuasive, the amount of systematic research on the modification of Type A behavior is remarkably sparse. Several recent reviews of this area (Gentry, 1978; Suinn, 1978, 1980; Chesney et al., 1981) reveal only a small number of studies which have postulated intervention strategies based on adequate conceptualizations of Type A behavior and which have then gone on to implement and evaluate these strategies. While other studies (for example, Rahe, Ward, & Hayes, 1979) have occasionally been cited as examples of attempts to modify Type A behavior in patients after myocardial infarction, the object of these studies has really been concerned with more general issues of counseling and rehabilitation and will not be dealt with in this chapter. Rather, it is proposed to review the studies that have specifically set out to modify Type A behavior, and to relate the conceptual basis of these studies to the theoretical model of Type A behavior previously put forward.

Perhaps the only study that has directed its attention specifically to survivors of myocardial infarction has been that of Friedman (1978). This is not in itself a problem, for there is no evidence to suggest that the principles applying to the modification of Type A behavior in healthy subjects or those with identified coronary risk should not generalize adequately to persons who have experienced and survived myocardial infarction. One might even speculate that the survivor of myocardial infarction would more readily accept a program aimed at modifying Type A behavior, because the presence of serious illness should act as a motivator for behavior change. This is, however, an issue more appropriately discussed under the heading of compliance and is dealt with later in the book.

3.1 Advice and Clinical Anecdote

Friedman and Rosenman (1974), in a presentation on Type A behavior aimed essentially at the nonprofessional person, suggested a series of strategies directed at its alteration. The focus of their program was twofold. The first related to personal awareness of Type A behaviors. This arose from the notion that while many people may exhibit Type A behaviors in a variety of situations, it is commonly reported that these behaviors are neither perceived as being Type A in character nor associated with feelings of undue stress or tension (Rosenman, 1978). In order to make people aware that they may be responding in a Type A fashion without recognizing it, Friedman and Rosenman (1974) produced a list of typical Type A behaviors extending across a variety of circumstances. These involved such examples as:

a. You make a habit of explosively accenting certain words in your ordinary speech.
b. You always move, walk, and eat rapidly.
c. You become quite irritated if you are stuck behind a slow car, if you have to wait in a queue, or if you are watching someone do something you know you could do faster.
d. You frequently try to think or do two or more things at the same time. For example, you continue to think about something on your mind while someone else is talking to you, you try to read while you eat, or eat while you drive, etc.
e. You attribute your success in good part to your ability to get things done faster than your fellow man and you are afraid to stop trying to do things faster and faster.

Indeed, even the briefest scan of this list alerts not only patients to the kinds of behaviors which have been identified as Type A, but also alerts clinicians to the kinds of behaviors which they may observe among those in their care, and which may later form the focus for intervention. Therefore, while the clinician who intends to become concerned with the modification of Type A behavior would do well to examine the various definitions of this phenomenon, a list such as that produced by Friedman and Rosenman (1974) serves the additional purpose of making such behaviors concrete and more readily identifiable within a clinical population.

The second phase of the program described by Friedman and Rosenman (1974) related to a set of exercises they designed to eliminate Type A behaviors whenever and wherever these were seen to occur. These strategies involved the deliberate imposition of alternative behaviors immediately a Type A behavior was identified, and emphasized self-management. Some examples of these strategies, again drawn from Friedman and Rosenman (1974), were:

a. Deliberately walk, eat, and talk slowly.
b. Monitor your time and become aware of the hours you spend in overtime work and in recreation. Decrease the former and increase the latter.
c. Discourage your Type A behaviors by penalizing yourself. For example, whenever you race through a yellow light at an intersection, force yourself to turn at the next corner and drive around the block.
d. Become aware of how often you glance at your wristwatch. Substitute some other action for this.

This is of course, closely akin to the long-standing behavioral strategy of response substitution (Rimm & Masters, 1979). Once more, examination of this list will be of considerable use to the clinician, as it provides a basis for the selection of appropriate alternative behaviors.

Useful as these strategies are, however, there are no empirical data which attest to their effectiveness. They are simply presented as exercises based on clinical observation and practice, and on the conceptualization of the Type A Behavior Pattern that Friedman and Rosenman (1974) held. Rosenman and Friedman (1977) presented data from a small pilot study involving 12 Type A men in a group program lasting 18 months. Groups were conducted by a therapist with a psychoanalytic background and intervention strategies were based on the notions espoused by Friedman and Rosenman (1974). There is little evidence to indicate the outcome of this program, though Chesney (1978) reported that anecdotal results arising from it were encouraging. The study does, however, present at least three difficulties that detract from its general utility in clinical practice. Firstly, the sample size was very small and there is no mention of a control group to allow proper evaluation. Secondly, there was little specific indication of the structure of the intervention strategies, save what has been mentioned above. The replication of such a study could not therefore be undertaken with any degree of exactness. Finally, there were no specific measures either of Type A behavior change or of alteration in risk of further myocardial infarction. Thus, the effectiveness of the program is difficult to judge in any quantitative way. One additional point deserves mention, as it bears on the general clinical utility of programs such as this. The duration of intervention was 18 months, and this seems excessively long. One wonders whether more effective strategies of intervention based on behavioral procedures might shorten this appreciably.

3.2   Systematic Studies of Type A Behavior Modification

The seminal work in this area has come from the studies of Suinn and his colleagues. This work, to which they have given the collective title Cardiac Stress Management Program (CSMP), was based on five premises (Suinn, 1980) considered essential in conceptualizing the process of Type A behavior modification. Firstly, they argued that stress management must be an early focus of intervention, because initial attempts to modify and reverse very ingrained patterns of Type A behavior may themselves lead to situational tension, and patients require the skills to combat this. Secondly, since time urgency and impatience were prominent components of Type A behavior, patients should experience relatively rapid changes in their behavior patterns so as to allay frustration which might arise from protracted intervention strategies. In order to achieve this they adopted a form of accelerated anxiety-management training previously developed by Suinn (1975, 1976). Thirdly, since persons with Type A behaviors frequently see these as equating with productivity and efficiency (Rosenman, 1978), any alternative behaviors or life-styles put forward should be seen as carrying the same advantages. Fourthly, behavioral retraining should emphasize a self-control model because Type A subjects may be reluctant to relinquish control of their own activities to others. Finally, it seemed most productive to give Type A persons the actual experience of producing alternative behaviors rather tham simply instructing in these. For this reason they devised a program of visuomotor behavior rehearsal (VMBR) (Suinn, 1972, 1976) where subjects rehearsed alternative behaviors under controlled conditions so that resulting stress could be effectively and rapidly alleviated.

In some respects, Suinn's conceptualization of the modification of Type A behavior seems similar to that originally advanced by Friedman and Rosenman (1974), with the emphasis on both awareness of Type A responses and the deliberate practice of alternative behaviors to these. The advance is, of course, that Suinn has refined this model and proposed concrete intervention strategies based on the principles of behavior modification.

Two studies have been undertaken to evaluate these strategies. In the first of these, Suinn (1975) investigated type A behavior modification in patients who had survived myocardial infarction. Ten patients were given five group sessions composed of both anxiety-management training and VMBR, and their progress was compared with a similar group of 10 subjects undergoing standard medical rehabilitation procedures. Outcome measures centered on indices of coronary risk, and in particular on serum lipid measures. Substantial decreases in both cholesterol and triglyceride levels were found for intervention subjects, both within the group (pre- versus post-test levels), and when the intervention group was compared with the control group. These findings were replicated in a further sample of 17 survivors of myocardial infarction who later undertook the intervention program (Suinn, 1980). However, while the intent of the program was to modify Type A behavior, no specific measures of this were used, and there is no way of telling whether changes in the behavior pattern were in fact achieved. Certainly, it is encouraging that intervention produced changes in coronary risk as indexed by cholesterol levels. Changes in Type A behavior, whether they were simultaneous or casual, can not, however, be inferred from these results.

In a subsequent study based on a similar conceptualization of Type A behavior modification, Suinn and Bloom (1978) used subjects drawn from a population of healthy volunteers. Behavioral intervention strategies closely similar to those employed in the previous study were offered to one group of these subjects, and outcome measures were compared with a control group to which no intervention program was offered. Each group consisted of seven subjects. The intervention program actually resulted in elevations in serum lipid levels among intervention subjects relative to control subjects. This, perhaps, says something of the differential effects of intervention between myocardial-infarction patients and ostensibly healthy subjects.

More importantly, however, measures of both Type A behavior and anxiety were employed in the study. Using these as outcome measures, it was found that intervention subjects showed significant decreases both in state and trait anxiety measures, and also in the *Speed and Impatience* and *Hard Driving* scales of the Jenkins Activity Survey, when compared with control subjects. This evidence is more pertinent to the issue, and provides some support for the contention that at least some aspects of Type A behavior are open to effective modification. The results, however, must be viewed cautiously for at least two reasons. Firstly the sample sizes were quite small and there were discrepancies between serum lipid results emerging from the first study (Suinn, 1975) and this subsequent study. Secondly, as Chesney et al. (1981) pointed out, the Jenkins Activity Survey total Type A scores were not significantly lower in the intervention group than in the control group and it is only this total score which has been found in epidemiological studies to be reliably predictive of myocardial infarction.

The other systematically evaluated approach to the modification of Type A behavior has arisen from the work of Roskies and her colleagues (1978, 1979), though the conceptual basis of this work differs markedly from that adopted by Suinn. The propositions upon which this work is based appear to be psychoanalytic in nature and involve the notion that Type A behavior arises from continued striving for maternal love and guilt over competition with the father. All other considerations aside, this appears to be something of a sexist notion of

Type A behavior in view of Waldron's (1978) evidence that women as well as men may manifest Type A attributes.

To examine this approach, Roskies, Spevack, Surkis, Cohen, and Gilman (1978) offered a program of 14 group sessions of psychotherapy run along psychoanalytic lines to a group of 13 healthy subjects with identified Type A behavior. The focus of these group sessions was to sensitize Type A persons to their apparent need to exert control over the environments within which they lived and to facilitate recognition of the maladaptive aspects of this situation. A second group of 12 healthy subjects, also with identified Type A behaviors, were taught in 14 group sessions to modify their Type A responses by means of standard stress management procedures. These procedures involved the continual monitoring of tension during daily life and the use of deep-muscle-relaxation exercises to counteract this tension. The group was identified as a behavior therapy group. A final and rather small group of six subjects consisted of patients with identified cardiovascular disease and was treated in the same way as the behavior therapy group.

Reductions in both cholesterol levels and systolic blood pressure were evident over the course of treatment for all groups; however, there were no significant differences between groups. A measure of psychological well-being, the General Health Questionnaire, which can be seen as a measure of state anxiety (Henderson, Byrne, & Duncan-Jones, 1981), also showed decreases over time for all groups. Once more, however, no standard measure of Type A behavior was consistently used. Subjects were asked for subjective self-reports of competitiveness and time urgency, and it was found that these self-reported attributes decreased over the course of treatment of all groups. Decreases were significantly greater for the behavioral group than for the psychotherapy group. In the absence of specific and recognized measures of Type A behavior, however, the results must be viewed tentatively.

Roskies et al. (1979) published a six month follow-up to their 1978 study in which it was found that changes in risk-factor levels for the behaviorally treated group with identified cardiovascular disease were significantly more enduring than changes in risk-factor levels for the group of healthy subjects treated with psychotherapy. Outcome measures for healthy subjects who were also treated behaviorally lay somewhere between these two groups.

Jenni and Wollersheim (1979) used volunteer subjects both with and without a history of cardiovascular disease, but with identified Type A behavior. These were assigned either to a behavioral intervention group emphasizing the restructuring of cognitions associated with Type A behavior, a stress management group involving the monitoring of tension and the use of procedures to counteract this, and a waiting-list control group. Each of the intervention groups involved six sessions. The cognitive-therapy group showed decreases in serum-cholesterol levels over the course of treatment relative to a minor increase in cholesterol in the waiting-list control group. There was, however, a substantial increase in cholesterol during the course of stress management, and this result, which clearly indicates an elevation in cardiovascular risk, is unexplained. Indices of both state and trait anxiety decreased over time in both intervention groups relative to the control group; however these changes were not enduring.

While the Structured Interview was used to assess subjects for Type A behavior at the beginning of the study, it was not readministered either after intervention or at follow-up. The Bortner scale (Bortner, 1969) was administered as a postintervention measure and Type A behaviors were not evident in the sample to any excessive degree. Direct comparisons between pretest and post-test measures can not, however, be made, because the scales differed appreciably between these two points of data collection.

Suinn (1981) quoted two unpublished studies that give some more support for the notion that Type A behavior is amenable to modification. Curtis (1974) used a collection of behavioral techniques, including stress management and autogenic training, as the basis for behavior modification in a group of healthy but Type A subjects. Comparison of intervention subjects with a control group also possessing Type A attributes revealed reductions among the former, in both cholesterol and triglyceride levels over the course of intervention, relative to the latter. Yarian (1976) used electromyographic biofeedback as a Type A intervention strategy and was able to demonstrate reductions in levels of frontalis muscle activity among Type A intervention subjects relative to Type A control subjects. In neither case, however, were explicit measures of Type A behavior used, and so once more it is not possible to attribute changes either in risk-factor levels (serum lipids) or tension levels (muscle activity) to preceding changes in Type A behavior.

The focus of a systematic study reported by Levenkron, Cohen, Mueller, and Fisher (1983) was a comparison of three methods (comprehensive behavior therapy emphasizing self-control procedures, group support but without specific behavioral procedures, and the provision of basic health information) for the modification of Type A behavior among healthy male volunteers. Pretreatment assessment included measures of self-reported Type A behavior together with scales of affective distress and measures of coronary-risk factors. Both behavior therapy and group support conditions involved weekly meetings of 90 minutes spread over eight consecutive weeks, while the final condition (information giving) involved a single two hour session. At follow-up one week after termination of each treatment condition, subjects involved in both behavior therapy and group support exhibited significantly lower scores on the Jenkins Activity Survey than did subjects in the information-only group. This pattern was evident also in self-reported reactions to a stress challenge test. Neither temporal changes nor differences between groups were, however, apparent for standard coronary-risk factors (heart rate, blood pressure, or blood fats). This study singled out anger and impatience, in particular, as useful targets for treatment.

Certainly, the most ambitious program of research yet to be undertaken in this area is that initiated under the direction of Friedman (1978). In this study, a cohort of 862 Type A males who had recently survived myocardial infarction were offered a variety of intervention programs aimed a modifying their Type A behaviors. Of these, 592 were randomly assigned to groups using a broad spectrum of intervention strategies, including self-observation and monitoring to increase awareness of Type A behavior, self-management of the environment, behavioral contracting, deep-muscle relaxation, anxiety-management training, and cognitive restructuring directed toward modifying Type A behavior. The remaining 270 were allocated to groups that emphasized traditional procedures of rehabilitation and include ''. . . conventional education regarding the need to reduce traditional risk factors and group psychotherapy to deal with problems of anxiety and depression'' (Surwit, et al. 1981).

Results of this large study have been encouraging, due in large part to a more than adequate sample size, the use of multiple measures of Type A behavior, and the prospective design of the investigaion. A two-year follow-up of patients taking part in the study has shown quite persuasively that Type A behavior is amenable to modification (Powell, Friedman, Thoresen, Gill, & Ulmer, 1984). Patients taking part in programs designed specifically to modify the behavior pattern were, after two years, significantly lower on Type A behavior as measured by self-report, the report of a spouse, and the report of a co-worker than were patients whose cardiac rehabilitation program was aimed at general issues and not-Type-A behavior. This result was also evident when the presence of Type A behavior was judged by independent raters viewing a videotape of the Structured Interview method of assessment. Of those involved in the Type A modification program, 17.9% showed reduction in multiple measures of Type A behavior; a further 29.4% on a single measure of the behavior pattern; only 21.5% failed to demonstrate any reduction, while 26.5% dropped out of the study.

The clinical importance of this program is evident, however, in a further report of the same cohort (Friedman et al., 1984) in which it can be seen that decreases in the rate of coronary events follow from reductions in the level of Type A behavior. The three-year cumulative recurrence rate for myocardial infarction among those receiving Type A behavior modification was, at 7.2%, significantly lower than the 13% found in those receiving a more medically orientated rehabilitation program. The implications of this finding are of considerable importance in the secondary prevention of myocardial infarction; however, the rull realization of this benefit must await the demonstration that modification of the Type A behavior pattern, when applied to those free of cardiac symptoms, results in significant reductions in the primary incidence of heart attack.

With the exception, then, of the work of Suinn and his colleagues (Suinn, 1975, 1981; Suinn & Bloom, 1978) and the extensive study of Friedman and his group, there has been little attempt either to spell out the conceptual basis for intervention strategies or to describe in sufficient detail the nature and course of the intervention processes undertaken. This is a critical deficiency as it allows neither the systematic replication of these studies nor translation of the intervention techniques into feasible strategies for routine clinical management of cardiac patients. This makes the adequate description of the intervention foci a crucial consideration in any future study of Type-A-behavior modification, whether it be experimental or clinical.

3.3   Future Directions in the Modification of Type A Behavior

While the studies quoted here may be criticized to varying degrees both on conceptual and methodological grounds, the results are nonetheless encouraging when viewed collectively. The evidence does point to the conclusion that deliberate strategies of behavior modification designed to counteract one or more of the attributes of the Type A behavior pattern can achieve useful reductions in coronary risk. Two questions remain unanswered, however, and require further consideration. The first concerns the specific aspects of Type A behavior which, if successfully modified, are likely to provide the greatest benefit in terms of reduced coronary morbidity and mortality. The second concerns the most appropriate strategies of intervention to modify these aspects of behavior.

It will be clear from the earlier sections of this chapter that Type A behavior is not a unitary phenomenon but is composed of a number of components (Jenkins & Zyzanski, 1982). With this in mind, one can see sense in the argument of Chesney et al. (1981), that the first step in any program of Type-A-behavior modification, whether it be experimental or clinical, is the specification of target behaviors. Two things need to be borne in mind in this respect. The first of these is that Type A behaviors, as already emphasized, take several forms and guises, and those aspects which are present in one individual need not necessarily be present in another. That is, people may differ considerably in terms of the Type A attributes they manifest. The second is that while Type A behavior contributes to coronary risk, it is rather less clear which components of Type A behavior are most damaging in this respect. All of this points to the need for individually tailored programs of Type-A-behavior modification designed to fit the specific demands of each individual patient. This assumes that the components of Type A behavior can and will be accurately measured as a precondition to modification, though there is some evidence of the kind quoted in Section 2 that measurement at least is a scientifically feasible exercise. The notion of individual programs also conflicts, to an extent, with the potential benefits arising from intervention with groups of patients. This is, *inter alia,* an economic argument, though within the context of a busy clinical practice it may be a very pertinent one.

Assuming then that we are at least able to specify for any individual those aspects of Type A behavior that are most prominent, it should be possible to list the available intervention strategies which might be brought to bear on their modification, whether these strategies have been examined specifically in relation to Type A subjects or whether they arise more generally from the literature in behavior modification.

3.3.1   Cognitive Strategies.   It seems clear that Type A behaviors as manifest responses arise from some predisposing set of cognitions or personal constructions of the environment. The most fundamental of the intervention strategies would, therefore, appear to be those based on the restructuring of these cognitions. The literature on cognitive restructuring within the general area of behavior modification is both large and conceptually well developed, and has provided consistently encouraging results in a variety of areas (Meichenbaum, 1977; Rimm & Masters, 1979). Jenni and Wallersheim (1978) reported their most promising results from the cognitive therapy group, and elements of cognitive restructuring can be discerned within the therapeutic strategies of Suinn (1981) and of Roskies et al. (1978), though in the latter study much of this is phrased within a psychoanalytic context. An examination of the range of strategies proposed by Friedman and his group also indicates a considerable reliance on those to do with cognitive restructuring. Clearly, the effective utilization of cognitive strategies will depend on the effective externalization and specification of what the offending cognitions may be. This is standard practice in any form of cognitive therapy. Having disclosed the internal dialogue hypothesized to cause people to respond to their environments in Type A ways, there is every reason to believe that those cognitive restructuring strategies which have been shown so successful in other areas, for example in the treatment of depression (Beck, 1967) and other emotional disorders (Meichenbaum, 1977), may be used equally effectively to modify cognitions that initiate and promote Type A behaviors.

3.3.2   Environmental Management.   A prominent aspect of the literature in this area has related to the ways in which social and cultural contexts might reinforce and maintain Type A behaviors once these are established (Rosenman, 1978). This presents a potential difficulty, as it might be surmounted only by social change on a large scale; and while this may be a desirable objective, it is infrequently a practical proposition. Environments can, of course, be changed in more modest ways. Chesney et al. (1981) point to the possibility of modifying home and work environments at an individual level without the need to consider social change on a grander scale. Modification of the social and occupational environments at this level may involve both monitoring, to discern those elements of the environment that are likely to reinforce Type A behaviors, and the use of deliberate strategies such as those suggested by Friedman and Rosenman (1974) to change these situations. This may be particularly useful in the work environment (Chesney & Rosenman, 1980), where the individual may be encouraged to exercise a degree of control over the amount of work undertaken, the amount of effort and time put into work, and the extent to which occupational considerations should override other activities such as those to do with leisure and recreation. However, in societies where the level of employment relates strongly to social and economic status, this should be undertaken with the patient's explicit acceptance that previously valued aspects of life-style may incur change. This may prove difficult given the common tendency to equate the time urgency and excess activity associated with Type A behavior with efficiency and productivity in one's work life.

3.3.3   Direct Behavior Change.   Type A behaviors take a wide variety of forms (see for example the lists produced in Friedman & Rosenman, 1974 and in Chesney et al., 1981), and though they come about as the result of situational determinants, their common characteristic is that they are overt and observable aspects of activity and life-style. Such behaviors, therefore, form a very apparent focus for intervention strategies.

Indeed, the thrust of Friedman and Rosenman's (1974) suggestions to Type A individuals to alter their behaviors was that they should quite deliberately adopt patterns of activity diametrically opposed to Type A behaviors. This area does, however, bear on the very mainstream of behavior therapy, and a wide range of well-established and evaluated techniques are available for the modification of maladaptive behaviors, whether they be Type A or other. Much of the emphasis of Suinn's (1981) work had to do with the immediate alteration of behaviors that were identified as Type A. This was based on the rationale that Type A subjects are most likely to respond favorably to procedures in which they can become experientially involved, and where relatively rapid changes, at least during the course of therapy, are likely to be evident. Two well-accepted procedures in behavior therapy, those of behavior rehearsal and response substitution, both using role-play methods, are important in this respect. Response substitution, or the deliberate initiation of an adaptive or neutral response where the situation might otherwise have produced a maladaptive response, is an established procedure in behavior therapy and has been used with success for a variety of disorders (Yates, 1975; Rimm & Masters, 1979). Within the context of Type-A-behavior modification, the patient would be encouraged to continually monitor personal behaviors for Type A responses. When these were likely to occur, the selection of an alternative non–Type A response, perhaps from a prearranged list, and the deliberate initiation of this behavior, would be practiced. When coupled with the technique of role play, where the patient is able to practice these response-substitution procedures in the absence of threat from the real environment, the process may form the basis for a useful strategy for the direct modification of Type A behaviors.

There is little evidence on the potential role of punishment procedures in the modification of Type A behavior. Friedman and Rosenman (1974), in their list of alternative behaviors, encouraged patients to deliberately punish themselves for behaving in a Type A fashion. The literature on punishment as an effective behavior modification strategy is, however, less and less encouraging (Rimm & Masters, 1979; Pechacek & McAlister, 1980). It is perhaps not surprising, then, that this avenue of Type-A-behavior modification has not been more extensively explored.

3.3.4   Time Management.   The prominence of time urgency within the Type-A-behavior pattern points to the potential effectiveness of time management in intervention. Individuals with this component of Type A behavior are typically poor managers of time, and this is perhaps most evident in their ". . . relatively chronic struggle to obtain an unlimited number of poorly defined things from their environment in the shortest period of time . . ." (Friedman, 1969). Procedures for the training of effective time management are, however, now available and have been evaluated (Lakein, 1973; Ferner, 1980). These procedures involve the monitoring and definition of areas where time management is ineffective, and the more rational allocation of available times to necessary tasks. Given the prominence of time urgency and its variety of manifestations within the overall Type-A-behavior pattern, it is likely that procedures for the retraining of time management will receive greater attention in future strategies of Type A intervention.

3.3.5   Hostility Management.   Overt hostility as a manifestation of Type A behavior is perhaps less prominent than one might expect given its repeated appearance in descriptions of the Type-A-behavior pattern (Herman et al., 1981), though these same authors reported that 62% of Type A subjects rated themselves as "aggressive," while Francis (1981) found that Type A subjects reported significantly higher levels of "state hostility" as evidenced on the Multiple Affective Adjective Check List than did their non–Type A colleagues. The procedures developed by Novaco (1975) for the management of anger and hostility, which emphasize self-monitoring, the restructuring of hostile cognitions, and the substitution of passive or neutral responses, would be well suited where hostility was found to be a prominent component of the presenting Type A pattern for any individual.

3.3.6   Stimulus Control.   Consideration of the direct modification of behaviors within the Type A pattern does raise one rather general issue in behavior therapy. The prevailing conceptions of the Type A pattern (Rosenman & Chesney, 1980) suggest that the overt and manifest behaviors are directly initiated by situational and environmental circumstances which may themselves be transient. That is, Type A behaviors seem, to an extent, to be under stimulus control. The area of stimulus control has been well documented in behavior therapy (Goldfried & Merbaum, 1973), and several of the intervention strategies alluded to previously may well have been discussed within the ambit of stimulus control. While no work has yet been done in this area, formalizations of intervention strategies based on the identification of situational determinants of Type A behavior, and the gradual dissociation of behaviors from their determinants, would seem to hold some conceptual promise.

3.3.7 Stress Management. As will be evident from earlier discussions, the appearance of distress or other affective disturbances as a consequence of Type A behaviors is still very much in debate (Byrne, 1981). Nonetheless, there is growing evidence that persons manifesting the Type A Behaviour Pattern will also experience and report signs of affective distress (Suinn, 1981). Indeed, as Suinn pointed out, the very process of attempting to modify Type A behaviors may lead to frustration and affective distress if the subject is unable to experience early success with behavior modification. The need to incorporate procedures for stress management into a comprehensive strategy of Type A behavior modification would, therefore, seem to be self-evident.

There is much to recommend Suinn's programs of anxiety management (Suinn, 1975; Suinn & Richards, 1971; Suinn & Bloom, 1978), to the extent that these are based both on well-researched processes of anxiety management and have been evaluated with cardiac patients. Progressive muscle relaxation clearly has an important role to play both in these programs and in others (Jenni & Wallersheim, 1978; Roskies et al., 1978). However, three cautions are advised in its use. The first is that, in isolation, relaxation is unlikely to be particularly effective, as it focuses on the consequences of Type A behaviors while doing little to modify these behaviors themselves. The second is that people with extreme degrees of Type A behavior may be unwilling to engage in the somewhat rigorous time demands of relaxation training in the absence of relatively immediate effects. Thus progressive muscle relaxation in the management of affective distress associated with Type A behavior is to be seen more as a component of intervention than as its central focus.

The final caution concerns the potentially damaging physiological effects of isometric procedures of muscle relaxation on the vulnerable myocardium in recent survivors of myocardial infarction. While the evidence suggests that ordinary procedures of muscle relaxation are unlikely to severely challenge the myocardial integrity of cardiac patients (Davidson et al., 1979) the use of more passive strategies for muscle relaxation must be advocated, at least in the early stages of recovery from myocardial infarction.

It should be borne in mind that where intervention is undertaken with the recent survivor of myocardial infarction, the affective picture may be confounded by the patient's immediate emotional responses to illness (Byrne, 1979; Byrne & Whyte, 1978). Thus, the pattern of affective distress evident in this period may not necessarily characterize the individual's state either before illness onset or in the long-term after. This does not detract from the potential value of the management of affective distress at this point, though the therapist should be aware that it is not necessarily Type A behavior that is being treated.

3.3.8   Psychophysiological Management.   There is little doubt that, at least under some circumstances, Type A behavior has definite psychophysiological consequences. These take the form of elevations both in heart rate and blood pressure (Steptoe, 1981), and might be seen to follow from pronounced adrenocortical activity (Frankenhaeuser et al., 1980). A range of behavioral techniques, including deep-muscle relaxation (Blanchard & Miller, 1977) and biofeedback of various kinds (Schwartz & Beatty, 1977) have been advocated for the control of this activity. A more detailed discussion of these techniques was given in Chapter 6 on the control of physiological risk factors after myocardial infarction, and further elaboration will not be given here.

It is worth bearing in mind, however, that if the cognitive and behavioral aspects of Type A behavior have been adequately addressed in any program of intervention, then the need to consider treatment at the physiological stage should have diminished. Indeed, this may even be seen as an instance of "putting the cart before the horse," and there would be some who would argue that if the psychophysiological consequences of Type A behavior are so pronounced as to pose a future threat, then they should be treated pharmacologically with the use of a beta blocking agent (Rosenman, 1983), while psychological management should simultaneously focus on the modification of events earlier in the process. This perhaps goes too far and denies the potential usefulness of behavioral techniques which might help to control physiological arousal, but it does underscore the primary importance of behavior modification at the level of cognitions and of Type A behaviors themselves.

3.4   Conclusions

While the literature which specifically relates behavior modification strategies to the alteration of Type A behavior is somewhat sparse, if taken along with the very much broader literature on behavior therapy (see Yates, 1975; Rimm & Masters, 1979, for reviews), one is encouraged that behavior therapy has much to offer in the area. Given the range of Type A behaviors and their antecedents and consequences, it is likely the most fruitful approach will not be to develop one single strategy for the modification of Type A behavior, but to draw from the wide variety of developed and evaluated procedures in behavior therapy so that the intervention strategy matches whatever is the identified focus of an individual's Type A pattern. This rationalization is, of course, entirely consistent with the tenets of scientific behavior therapy. It underscores the point that Chesney et al. (1981) made concerning the correct selection of targets for Type A behavior modification. It also implies that Type-A-behavior modification will be more effective when tailored to the presenting problems of single individuals than when given to small collections of perhaps diverse individuals in groups. This is a difficult argument to deal with because group work presents a more economical approach to clinical management of this kind. There may also be distinct advantages in managing some aspects of Type A behavior in groups in the sense that such procedures as behavior rehearsal and role play can be more easily contrived where a small number of people are available. The practicability of individual versus group treatment may ultimately rest with the numbers of Type A patients in any single clinical unit.

The absence of adequate prospective studies on Type-A-behavior modification provides little evidence to allow comment on the maintenance of Type-A-behavior change. Complete reviews of studies pertinent to other areas of coronary risk—for example, smoking (Pechacek & McAlister, 1981), indicate that while behavior change might be quite effective in the short term, its endurance is less than encouraging. While Schachter (1981) has recently challenged these conclusions, there does seem some cause for concern that the maintenance of Type-A-behavior change may pose problems. This, in turn, recommends the meticulous follow-up of patients after Type A intervention, and the application of maintenance strategies when these appear to be necessary. The potential for social and cultural facilitation of Type A behaviors, particularly within some groups where occupational factors are of a high priority, makes this an even more important consideration.

The several steps necessary in Type-A-behavior modification have been summarized by Chesney et al. (1981), and some additions to this summary provide a working clinical guide for practice in this area of behavioral medicine. These steps are:

a. The assessment of the individual patient and the identification of targets for intervention, whether these be overt Type A behaviors, their cognitive antecedents or their affective and physiological consequences;

b. The selection and implementation of appropriate intervention strategies, whether these be based on previous work on the modification of Type A behavior or drawn from the broader armamentarium of behavior therapy;

c. The systematic measurement of Type A behaviors before, during, and after intervention;

d. The simultaneous measurement of changes in associated coronary risks—for example, blood pressure, levels of serum lipids, and the like;

e. Adequate follow-up of each individual, with careful attention to the possible need for maintenance strategies.

If these steps are followed, then there is every reason to believe that Type A behavior and its associated states, insofar as they consitute risks of further coronary disease, may be effectively managed in the cardiac patient.

CHAPTER 8

Compliance and the Cardiac Patient

1. INTRODUCTION

Compliance with health-care instructions is an issue of universal significance in medicine. The recency of this recognition is evident in the great expansion of published material on compliance that has appeared over the past 10 years (Haynes, 1979). While the initial impetus for this work (and perhaps that which remains primary) was the desire to improve therapeutic effectiveness across a broad range of conditions, opinions are now being raised that the economics of health care might be better served by improvements in compliance rates than by the detection and treatment of new cases, at least for some categories of illness (Masur, 1981).

Research into patient compliance has traditionally been directed at the three broad areas of rates of compliance, determinants of compliance, and the modification of compliance behavior in the direction of its improvement. Issues of both prevention and treatment behaviors have been addressed and the range of illnesses forming the foci for investigation has been extensive. Problems of compliance with treatment instructions among cardiac patients, particularly those receiving active therapy for hypertension, have been prominent in this literature. It is clear that while the problems of compliance among cardiac patients have formed a rich area of investigation in their own right, the principles governing their appearance and modification are essentially the same as those relating to compliance behavior in general (Haynes, Taylor, & Sackett, 1979).

1.1 Definitions of Compliance

Compliance exists where the patient faithfully and accurately adheres to instructions regarding the prevention or treatment of an illness state, given by a physician or other health-care worker. The behaviors which make up this somewhat global concept may be as simple and apparently convenient as the once-daily taking of medication or as complex and time consuming as a structured daily exercise program or a diet enhancing or restricting intake of specific nutrient substances. The most prominent reason underlying the rise of this area to such prominence in health-care research is of course the failure by many patients to adhere to medical instructions, either in the short or long term (Haynes et al., 1979) and the subsequent effects which this has on the prevention and treatment of illness. Estimates by these authors indicate that when averaged across all categories bearing on compliance with medical instructions only, around 50% of patients can be seen to accurately commence the behaviors required for prevention or treatment and to follow these through to their prescribed conclusion.

Definitions of compliance or failure to comply are frequently operationalized in terms of specific measures of compliance behavior. Thus, compliance may be defined as occurring if a patient with hypertension completes a course of medication or if a smoker at risk of coronary heart disease attends a smoking cessation program through to its end. Compliance might also be defined as having occurred if a particular outcome of prevention or treatment is reached, so that a patient placed on a cholesterol-lowering diet might be assumed to have complied if levels of serum cholesterol are acceptably reduced at the conclusion of treatment.

1.2   Measures of Compliance

Since both definitions of compliance and data on compliance rates rely strongly on the nature and accuracy of measures used, this aspect of compliance behavior has been closely researched. It is not the intention of this section to exhaustively review the material on the measurement of compliance because a number of recent reviews (see, e.g., Gordis, 1979; or Masur, 1981) have given very careful consideration to the issues involved. Rather, the section aims to look briefly at measures of patient compliance which may be conveniently applied within the clinical setting, with particular respect to the cardiac patient.

According to Masur (1981), measures of compliance are typically discussed under the following categories:

a. *Provider prediction*—where those professionals providing health care instructions also judge the extent to which their patients will comply with those instructions. There is general agreement that health-care providers are poor predictors of patient compliance. Caron and Roth (1968) in a study of compliance with medication regimes among patients with peptic ulcer reported that physicians were unable to estimate their patients' drug intake to a degree more accurate than chance. The most consistent error appeared to be that of overestimating patient compliance. In a study involving a more heterogeneous group of patients, Mushlin and Appel (1977) found that physicians could predict only 35% of patients who were detected by other means as being noncompliant with medication intake.

b. *Patient self-report*—where the measure of compliance comprises the patients' individual reports of health behaviors. This is the most commonly used method of assessing patient compliance; and despite some doubts as to the accuracy of patient self-report, there is encouraging evidence that it may realistically reflect compliance. While patients who report themselves as compliant when in fact they are not are difficult to detect, there is some evidence (Haynes, Taylor, Sackett, Gibson, Bernholz, & Mukherjee, 1980) to suggest that self-report compliance with antihypertensive medication consumption correlates quite highly with more objective measures of compliance behavior. A study of compliance with dietary instructions among cardiac patients (Remmell, Gorder, Hall, & Tillotson, 1980) suggested that the accuracy of self-reported compliance could be enhanced by the simple provision of a dietary record sheet given to the patient prior to the commencement of treatment.

c. *Medication measurements*—in which the responsible clinician directly monitors the intake of medication (this procedure can be extended to include the direct observation of such behaviors as smoking or dietary intake, or the direct recording of participation in exercise or rehabilitation groups by the clinician involved with the care of the patient). Evidence in support of this measure is generally encouraging (Masur, 1981); medication counts have been found to correlate at acceptably high levels with more direct measures with drug intake among patients with hypertension (Haynes et al., 1980), however Gordis (1979) warns that the disappearance of medication from the container is not a foolproof indication that it has been consumed by the patient.

d. *Clinical outcome*—where the level of compliance with treatment is inferred from the success or failure of the therapeutic program. As Masur (1981) points out, this inference is logically inconsistent since factors other than the treatment regime may impinge on the success or failure of the clinical outcome. Consequently, this measure of compliance is infrequently used in systematic studies.

e. *Direct chemical analysis*—in which specific changes in biological chemistry known to reflect compliance with particular therapeutic strategies are objectively tested for. In the case of medication, this may take the form either of the addition of specific detectable tracer substances to the drug or of specific postingestion measures of levels of the drug or its metabolites in the blood or urine (Hodge, Lynch, Davison, Knight, Sinn, & Carey, 1979). Chemical investigation may also be used, however, to monitor other forms of compliance behavior. It is now possible, for example, to detect compliance with smoking-cessation programs by means of chemical analyses of carbon-monoxide attachment to hemoglobin or the presence of thiocyanate levels in the saliva (Pechacek & McAlister, 1980). Methods of direct chemical analysis are, therefore, perhaps the most objective tests of compliance behavior. They are, however, also time consuming and potentially expensive, and the benefits in relation to costs may not be wholly justified, particularly where less intrusive methods of acceptable accuracy (patient self-report coupled with clinical interview) may suffice.

1.3   Rates of Compliance among Cardiac Patients

Sackett and Snow (1979) have provided a comprehensive overview of rates of compliance in relation to a broad spectrum of illnesses. From the evidence they present it is clear that compliance ranges widely according to the nature of the illness, the duration of the treatment, the inconvenience or discomfort associated with the therapy, the demographic characteristics of the sample, and the kind of measure used to assess compliance. It might be thought that anxiety associated with a diagnosis of a cardiac condition would act as a powerful motivator, both to adhere to medical instructions and to alter behaviors increasing the risk of further illness. In fact, compliance among cardiac patients portrays the same alarming attitudes to personal responsibility for health care as does adherence to medical instructions arising from other kinds of illnesses.

Studies of compliance in cardiac patients can be conveniently divided into two categories, the first dealing with essentially asymptomatic conditions such as high blood pressure, the second to do with conditions where symptoms are more apparent—for example, treatment following myocardial infarction. Compliance with instructions designed to alleviate asymptomatic conditions is notoriously low. With regard to the cardiac patient, two conditions, both of which are established risk factors for primary and recurrent myocardial infarction serve to illustrate this. Noncompliance with antihypertension treatment regimes has been exhaustively cited. Briggs, Lowenthal, Cirksena, Price, Gibson, and Flamenbaum (1975) evaluated compliance during beta-blocker (propranolol) therapy for the treatment of hypertension among uremic patients receiving intermittent outpatient hemodialysis. Their results lead to the comment that ''noncompliance occurred with remarkable frequency'' and this failure to adhere to antihypertensive medication instructions was associated with persistently poor control of blood pressure. When patients were divided among those who were compliant and those who were not, blood-pressure control was significantly better in patients adequately adhering to the therapeutic regime. Reported rates of compliance with antihypertensive medication range from only 16% among black women attending a family-planning clinic in South Africa (Hall, Hall, & Gold, 1976) to 97% among employed adults on a single white-collar work site in the United States (Alderman & Schoenbaum, 1975). Dropout rate from programs of antihypertensive medication appears to be concentrated in the first year of treatment (Abernethy, 1976) with total noncompliance rates of up to 48% being reported during this period (Rudd, Tul, Brown, Davidson, & Bostwick, 1979). Noncompliance with these programs is more pronounced among those for whom a satisfactory therapeutic effect is not immediately apparent (Silas, Tucker, & Smith, 1980). However, where satisfactory control of blood pressure can be demonstrated, long-term compliance with medication over a period of one to five years can be expected from between 75% and 80% of patients (Aberg, Hadstrand, & Lithell, 1980; Lovell, Stephens, Thomson, & Ulman, 1976; Stamler et al., 1975).

The modification of cigarette smoking as a coronary-risk factor may also be used to illustrate the failure to comply among those at risk of coronary heart disease but without conspicuous symptoms. In this case, however, the measure of compliance is not the commission of a particular behavior such as medication taking, but the cessation of smoking behavior. Thus, compliance is to an extent confounded with outcome. As can be seen from Chapter 6, a range of strategies for smoking cessation or reduction can achieve quite acceptable results in the short term. Failure to comply is, however, evident in two aspects of the smoking-cessation process. The first occurs during treatment, where dropout rates for smoking-cessation programs or poor attendance over a sequence of treatment sessions may reach unacceptably high levels (McAlister, 1975). The second occurs following termination of formal smoking-cessation programs, where continued compliance with smoking-cessation strategies and instructions frequently lapses, with the result that smoking cessation rates in around 70% of those who were initially successful in stopping smoking revert to baseline rates of smoking within three months of a treatment program (Pechacek & McAlister, 1981). This latter phenomenon has resulted in a degree of research interest in methods to enhance continued compliance with smoking-cessation strategies following initial success.

In general, community adherence to population programs designed to reduce coronary-risk factors en masse can be relatively good, as evidenced by the North Karelia project in Finland (World Health Organization, 1981). Compliance at an individual level with strategies designed to reduce coronary-risk factors can, however, be disappointingly low (Haynes et al., 1979).

It has often been assumed that the appearance of symptoms, especially those as dramatic as myocardial infarction, might act as a powerful motivating force both for compliance with specific treatment instructions and for the modification of behaviors assumed to be associated with risk of further illness. As has been noted, however, evidence relating to compliance with strategies for rehabilitation following myocardial infarction does not unconditionally support this assumption.

Bruce, Frederick, Bruce, and Fischer (1976) introduced 547 men and 56 women, 84.5% of whom had clinical manifestations of coronary heart disease, into a cardiopulmonary rehabilitation program. This involved sessions of graded physical training requiring between 30 and 60 minutes of activity on three mornings a week. The length of the program was indefinite, and while individual sessions were self-directed, the program was under continuous medical supervision. Some 58% of patients failed to comply (dropped out) over a period of around 8.6 months, while the remaining patients continued to be active in the program (that is, complying with exercise instructions) for up to 22 months. In a similarly large program involving exercise rehabilitation for survivors of myocardial infarction (Oldridge et al., 1983), 46.5% of an initial cohort of 678 men who were originally enrolled in the program either failed to complete it or complied inadequately with its overall content. Data reported by Carmody, Senner, Malinow, and Matarazzo (1980) suggest that where rehabilitation exercise programs for cardiac patients extend over prolonged periods of time, the greatest risk of dropout occurs during the first three months.

Results not unlike these have recently emerged from programs emphasizing a psychotherapeutic orientation to cardiac rehabilitation. In probably the first systematic program of its type (Ibrahim et al., 1974) it was reported that 84% of survivors of myocardial infarction initially agreed to participate in a series of psychotherapeutically oriented rehabilitation meetings. These were organized as weekly sessions of one and a half hours duration and extended over 50 weeks. Of the initial cohort, only 15.5% failed to comply completely by discontinuing attendance at weekly sessions. Average weekly individual attendance at sessions was, however, only 69% suggesting that while some individuals remain in the rehabilitation program for its entire course, their compliance along the way is by no means perfect.

By contrast to the protracted program of rehabilitation offered by Ibrahim and his colleagues, a study by Rahe, Ward, and Hayes (1979) investigated psychotherapeutic rehabilitation for survivors of myocardial infarction involving only six sessions of intervention. However, while all patients had given a verbal contract to attend all six sessions in a series, it was found that between 65% and 77% of patients (depending on the nature of the group) only were able to attend four or more of the intervention sessions. A study by Langosch, Seer, Brodner, Kallinke, Kulick, and Heim (1982) also emphasized relatively brief psychological intervention following myocardial infarction; however, intervention strategies in this instance were more concretely behavioral than strategies described by either Ibrahim or by Rahe. Even so, between 18% and 20% of patients failed to complete the whole course of cardiac rehabilitation and, therefore, to comply with strategies aimed at improving health.

It is clear then that the cardiac patient is not unique as a noncomplier with medical instructions. Whether the instructions relate to the treatment of asymptomatic conditions such as hypertension (either as primary or secondary prevention), or to conditions where the symptomatic state is both apparent and pronounced, such as that which follows myocardial infarction, a noticeable percentage of patients will fail to adhere to advice, instruction, and specific strategies designed to alleviate symptoms and prolong life. There is in addition evidence to indicate that those failing to comply with such instructions are at greater risk of future illness, whether revived or not, than those who accurately adhere to directions given to them by their physicians or others involved in their health care. The implications of this for strategies designed to enhance compliance are clear-cut.

2.   THE ENHANCEMENT OF COMPLIANCE

2.1   Determinants of Compliance Among Cardiac Patients

Factors influencing compliance behavior have been extensively reviewed (Haynes et al., 1979; Masur, 1981) and this large material will not be dealt with at length in this section. It is clear from the evidence on determinants of compliance, however, that those factors that hold true for compliance in general are broadly applicable to compliance among cardiac patients. Masur (1981) has suggested that determinants of compliance may be characterized under the headings of demographic attributes of the individual, features of the treatment program, and psychosocial variables.

As far as the first of these is concerned, the evidence is equivocal, and neither age, sex, marital status, nor social class have been consistent predictors of compliance behavior (Masur, 1981). In the particular case of the cardiac patient, this conclusion seems to hold, with the exception that older patients appear to adhere more closely to antihypertensive medication instructions than do younger patients (Peitzman, Bodison, & Ellis, 1982), whereas younger patients appear more likely to reject medical advice while in the coronary-care unit and to discharge themselves prematurely (Baile, Brinker, Wachspress, & Engel, 1979).

In a general sense, aspects of the treatment strategy present more clear-cut determinants on compliance with health-care instructions; the more complex the demands of a health-care strategy, the less likely it is that patients will comply with the directions associated with that strategy (Masur, 1981). Thus, the modification of coronary-risk factors such as cigarette smoking or Type A behavior, where it is necessary to change complex patterns of activity, are less likely to be met with patient compliance than are treatment strategies involving the relatively more simple act of consuming a pill. Similarly, the less convenient a health-care strategy, the more likely it is that patients will fail to comply with that strategy, though this may be somewhat modified by the nature of the treatment. Inconvenience was given as one of the principal reasons for failing to comply with an exercise program following an episode of coronary heart disease (Andrew et al., 1981) while self-reported convenience of consuming antihypertensive medication appears to have little effect on compliance with pill consumption among patients with identified hypertension (Sackett et al., 1975). Duration of treatment has an almost certain effect, at least on compliance with antihypertensive medication, with patients requiring treatment of long duration being far less likely to comply with medication taking than patients requiring shorter periods of treatment (Gillum, Neutra, Stason, & Solomon, 1979). These authors also reported that patients with less-severe illness were less likely to comply with treatment instructions than patients with more severe illness. This is consistent with the general speculation (Carnahan & Nugent, 1975) that notoriously poor compliance behavior with the treatment of hypertension as a coronary-risk factor is closely related to the asymptomatic nature of the condition.

These factors are, of course, mitigated by the nature of the communication between health-care givers and health-care consumers. Thus, it has been repeatedly shown that efforts to improve communication regarding medical instructions both from the point of view of its formulation by the health-care giver and its reception by the consumer also act to enhance overall levels of compliance with treatment (Ley, 1982; Ley & Morris, 1984).

Within the context of management, psychosocial influences on compliance are perhaps the most interesting, for they present a clear focus for intervention and modification. A prominent approach to this has been to emphasize the interaction between the provider and the consumer of health care (Stone, 1979). This has been reinforced by a recent and extensive review of relevant studies (Ley, 1982) in which it was concluded that dissatisfaction among patients with communication between them and their health-care providers is widespread and leads, in turn, to poor compliance with health-care instructions. There is certainly evidence that this holds for the cardiac patient, both with regard to the treatment of hypertension among patients at risk of coronary-heart disease (Zacest, Barrow, O'Halloran, & Wilson, 1981) and among patients undergoing rehabilitation programs following a clinical episode of coronary heart disease (Soloff, 1980). It is fair to conclude then, that failure to comply with health-care instructions among cardiac patients is, at least in part, a function of their dissatisfaction with patterns of interaction and communication with their health-care providers. This may, of course, reflect as much a difficulty arising from patients as from their clinicians.

Perhaps the most comprehensive model examining the role of psychosocial and behavioral influences in the determination of compliance behavior is the Health Belief Model (Becker & Maiman, 1975). This holds that the probability of complying with medical instructions, be they therapeutic or preventive, is a function of a set of individual beliefs regarding the nature of the illness in question. These beliefs arise from individual perceptions of the discomfort, severity, and threat associated with a particular illness (which are then modified by the demographic attributes of the individual) as well as from the operation of specific individual personality patterns, and prevailing attitudes regarding the illness held both by close social groups and by society at large. While the model is undeniably a complex one, it has allowed the prediction of compliance behavior to a reasonable extent for a wide variety of illness conditions (Masur, 1981).

Johnson (1979) found in a survey of hypertensive patients attending a treatment clinic that the most prevalent beliefs regarding high blood pressure and its treatment had to do with concern with treatment efficacy and fear of unpleasant side effects. Attention to these health beliefs by the clinician would, it was suggested, act to enhance compliance with antihypertensive medication taking. Beliefs regarding the doubtful efficacy of antihypertensive medication and their effect on compliance have also been reported by Nelson, Stason, Neutra, Solomon, and McArdle (1978).

The use of the Health Belief Model to predict compliance behavior among cardiac patients has not been widespread; its application has had largely to do with compliance with treatment strategies for high blood pressure among those at risk of coronary heart disease. The onset of myocardial infarction, with its pronounced symptoms set within a well-known context of distinct and prevalent community attitudes, is likely to have a unique effect on beliefs regarding outcome and treatment. Earlier chapters of this book deal at some length with the nature of psychological responses to myocardial infarction and the relationship which these bear to outcome. This work has not addressed itself specifically to the prediction of compliance behavior among survivors of myocardial infarction; however, it is likely that because many of the elements composing the Health Belief Model have already been specified and measured for patients recovering from heart disease, the Health Belief Model may provide a useful framework for future studies concerned with the acceptance of and adherence with treatment programs—in particular those of rehabilitation following heart attack.

2.2   The Modification of Compliance Behavior

Given the widespread failure of patients to comply with medical instructions, it is not surprising that a considerable amount of research into compliance has to do with the development and evaluation of strategies concerned with its improvement. While a recent review (Dunbar, Marshall, & Hovell, 1979) suggested that these approaches may be described under the general headings of educational, organizational, and behavioral strategies, the literature documenting compliance enhancement in cardiac patients does not allow such distinct compartmentalization. Moreover, the evidence is drawn largely from studies documenting the enhancement of compliance with treatments attending to the control of coronary-risk factors among people without conspicuous coronary heart disease. Few studies have addressed the issue of compliance enhancement among survivors of myocardial infarction. There is, of course, no reason to believe that the principles arising from these data cannot be generalized to the modification of compliance behavior among survivors of myocardial infarction.

The available literature suggests that several strategies, either singly or in combination, hold some promise for improving compliance behavior among cardiac patients, whether these be patients at risk or patients in whom the onset of coronary heart disease has occurred. These may be discussed under the following headings:

(a) *Patient education strategies*—where compliance is improved by means of the provision of detailed but understandable information about the illness, treatment, or both. Espinosa de Restrepo (1981), reporting on the results of a four-year study of treatment for hypertension, claimed that the most important strategy for improving compliance was the provision for patients of educational material regarding high blood pressure and its treatment, particularly where this was reinforced by regular contact with paramedical personnel. A study by Webb (1980), however, which compared the effectiveness of educational strategies at various levels of intensity on the compliance of hypertensive patients, found that intensive education aimed directly at the salient issue was no more effective in improving compliance than was more casual education carried out during regular visits to the family physician. This was also shown to be the case for a group of obese patients enrolled in a weight-reduction program following a survived myocardial infarction (Wright, Wood, & Hale, 1981), where it was shown that an intensive program of nutrition education was no more effective in maintaining compliance than a program involving only the provision of simple written information. By contrast, intensive educational programs regarding both the illness and its treatment have been shown noticeably to improve compliance in rehabilitation programs among patients recovering from both myocardial infarction (Pozen, Stechmiller, Harris, Smith, Fried, & Voigt, 1977) and cardiothoracic surgery (Linde & Janz, 1979). Indeed, in the latter study, it was shown that the more professionally qualified the educator, the more effective was the education program in improving compliance. Educational strategies may, therefore, have some use in modifying compliance behavior among cardiac patients, particularly where these patients have already experienced myocardial infarction. Care must be taken, however, to tailor the educational program to the ability of the patient to understand it (Ley & Morris, 1984).

(b) *Regular patient follow-up*—where compliance with treatment is improved by way of structured, regular, and sometimes frequent monitoring by the healthcare provider. Fletcher, Appel, and Bourgeois (1975) randomly assigned hypertensive patients just beginning treatment, either to a group for whom regular follow-up contact was arranged, or to a group left to arrange follow-up contact for themselves. Significantly more patients in the former group than in the latter demonstrated compliance with the treatment strategy; however, these differences appeared to equalize over a period of about five months. Similar results, at least in the short term, have been reported by Glanz, Kirscht, and Rosenstock (1981). A study by Takala, Niemella, Rosti, & Sievers (1979) delayed the introduction of regular follow-up until patients, by their own behavior, had been identified as noncompliant with regard to antihypertensive medication. The provision of regular follow-up for these patients significantly improved their compliant behavior over time, with a subsequent improvement in levels of blood pressure. Patient follow-up may, therefore, facilitate improvement of compliance behavior among cardiac patients. However, there are indications (Fletcher et al., 1975) that compliance-improving strategy may need to be maintained over time in order to maintain compliance itself.

(c) *Patient self-monitoring*—where patients themselves are charged with the monitoring of both the implementation and success of the treatment strategy, with the added obligation, in some studies, to report results of this monitoring at regular intervals to the health-care provider. Baile and Engel (1978) used behavioral self-monitoring as part of a package to improve compliance among a group of patients recovering from myocardial infarction who had previously demonstrated noncompliant behaviors. Rates of compliance increased in all patients following implementation of the program; however, since there was no control group, it is difficult to say either that the package was in itself uniquely effective relative to attention alone or that the element of self-monitoring contributed a unique effect to the outcome. Attention to study design has, however, allowed more clear-cut inferences to be drawn from other work evaluating self-monitoring to enhance compliance among hypertensives. Haynes et al. (1976) found that self-monitoring of both blood pressure and medication consumption was an effective way of improving compliance with antihypertensive medication among patients with uncontrolled hypertension who had previously demonstrated noncompliant behavior. This finding has been echoed in the results of Nessman, Carnahan, and Nugent (1980), where the benefits of compliance are also to be seen in terms of reductions in blood pressure. Gelman and Nemati (1981) have suggested that this strategy for improving compliance with antihypertensive treatment may be most effective where self-monitoring, at least of blood pressure, can be achieved simply and without the need for complicated equipment. There is, of course, general support for the efficacy of behavioral self-monitoring in the control of health and other behaviors (Rimm & Masters, 1979), and it is possible that further systematic research may confirm the utility of this procedure for improving compliance among cardiac patients experiencing difficulty in adhering to medical instructions.

(d) *Social support and counseling*—where the aid of either significant others or of a health professional is enlisted in order to persuade the patient of the need for compliance. The mobilization of family support has been successfully used to enhance compliance among patients undertaking a cholesterol-lowering diet program (Witschi, Singer, Wu-Lee, & Stare, 1978). Moreover, the support of peer groups has been found useful in the maintenance of compliance with smoking cessation strategies. Webb (1980) reported, however, that support from a professional counselor was of little additional use to patients experiencing difficulty in complying with a program of antihypertensive medication relative to routine support given by the family physician. The mobilization of social support may, therefore, be a less effective means of improving compliance behavior among cardiac patients than among patients with other illnesses (Dunbar et al., 1979).

2.3   Overview

Documentation of noncompliance among cardiac patients, whether these be patients at risk or those in whom disease is evident, has been widespread in the recent literature—though studies of the improvement of compliance among cardiac patients have been much more sparse. Studies have concentrated, to a degree, on compliance among patients at risk of myocardial infarction, in contrast to a relative scarcity of studies on the modification of compliance among patients who have already experienced a myocardial infarction. Within the former category, the issue of noncompliance and its improvement among patients with hypertension has been a prominent focus for research. Therefore, while the principles of compliance improvement may possibly generalize from patients at risk to patients with identified coronary heart disease, the indications for management among the latter are rather less well substantiated.

Where compliance-improvement strategies are documented, these appear to concentrate more on interventions involving educational and organizational procedures than on those involving behavioral techniques. The conspicuous exception to this concerns the self-monitoring strategies, where more uniquely behavioral principles can be seen to operate.

Dunbar et al. (1979), having reviewed studies on the modification of compliance behavior in general, conclude that ". . . the independent effect of these [behavioral] strategies on compliance has not been dramatic." They go on to advise that where compliance-enhancement procedures—particularly those based on behavioral principles—are used, they are most likely to be effective when presented in a package consisting of multiple strategies. Failure to comply with medical instructions continues to be a difficulty among cardiac patients, and the onset of myocardial infarction does not appear to improve compliance to any pronounced degree. The clinical management of noncompliance among these patients is not at present guided by any single cohesive model. It may ultimately reduce to the intelligent selection of a package of individual strategies tailored to fit the specific needs of an individual patient.

CHAPTER 9

Psychological Intervention With the Cardiac Patient: An Integration

1. THE ISSUE

Evidence on the psychophysiology of cardiovascular activation (Surwit et al., 1982) irrefutably supports the case that behavior and personality can directly influence cardiac functioning. With particular reference to the evidence associating psychophysiological factors with sudden cardiac death, Lown and his colleagues (Lown et al., 1980) claimed:

> A considerable body of evidence indicates that the higher nervous system modifies electrical activity of the heart and may trigger sudden death.

They went on to advise:

> The involvement of psychiatrists, psychologists, and cardiologists in a multidisciplinary approach to managing patients at risk for sudden death from ventricular fibrillation is yielding significant insights and prolonging their lives.

These sentences, generalized to all survivors of myocardial infarction, concisely encapsulate the theme of the present book.

The preceding chapters draw on published evidence in order to document an argument embodying three sequential elements. Firstly, psychological and behavioral responses to myocardial infarction have been measured and appear to fit into characteristic patterns. Secondly, these patterns of responses are associated, probably causally, with patterns of outcome following myocardial infarction. Thirdly, psychological and behavioral intervention aimed at modifying apparently maladaptive patterns of response to myocardial infarction, together with psychological and behavioral interventions directed toward the modification of risk factors associated with the primary onset of the illness, may act to reduce prolonged disability and discomfort after heart attack and increase chances of survival.

2. MEDICAL CARE AND PSYCHOLOGICAL INTERVENTION

Responsibility for the management of the cardiac patient following myocardial infarction has traditionally fallen to the physician. The correctness of this role can not be challenged; myocardial infarction is fundamentally a physiological dysfunction requiring the monitoring, restabilization, and rebuilding of a complex biological system. To deny the medical focus of management would be foolhardy.

It is now clear, however, that in a substantial number (probably the majority) of cases, medical care alone is insufficient to satisfy the full range of needs evident among cardiac patients who have recently survived myocardial infarction. In the short term, most survivors of myocardial infarction experience pronounced and frequently unnecessary emotional distress. In the longer term, these same patients may adopt behaviors, perhaps in response to this distress, that are at odds with the achievement of recovery and rehabilitation. It is also evident that behaviors existing prior to the onset of illness, which may have been seen to contribute to the initial episode of myocardial infarction, extend into the period after the illness event and may place the patient at risk of a further heart attack. It is certainly clear from the evidence discussed in Chapter 5 that the provision of psychological-intervention programs after myocardial infarction, designed to facilitate both recovery and rehabilitation, significantly enhances outcome assessed along a range of criteria, when compared with outcomes following the provision of medical care alone. The overriding clinical issue facing the cardiological team should, therefore, not be whether psychological intervention in its various forms should be contemplated, but how it should be integrated into the overall management program of the cardiac patient.

3. THE ORGANIZATION OF PSYCHOLOGICAL
INTERVENTION

The structuring of psychological intervention within a cardiological setting raises three issues of procedure. The first has to do with whether psychological intervention is provided as a consultative service that may be called upon only when the physician judges it to be necessary, or whether all survivors of myocardial infarction should be routinely seen at least once (for screening) by a clinician whose designated role it is to organize and provide psychological intervention. The second is concerned with whether such intervention, routine or otherwise, is provided on an individual or group basis. The third relates to the stage of illness at which psychological intervention may be most conveniently and effectively commenced.

The empirical evidence guiding decisions in these areas is not abundant.

Clearly, not all patients experiencing myocardial infarction will respond with unwarranted emotional distress or with behaviors likely to impede the course of recovery and rehabilitation. Nonetheless, as Doehrman (1977) has pointed out, temporary disruption of normal psychological and social functioning is to be observed in most patients, while long-standing disturbances will occur in a significant minority. Mayou, Williamson, and Foster (1978a) have cautioned that psychosocial disruption among survivors of myocardial infarction is probably far more widespread than is commonly recognized and that this form of disability has often been neglected by those involved in the care of the cardiac patient. The evidence on psychological intervention following myocardial infarction (see Chapter 5) is consistent in its support of the benefits to be gained from this intervention. These considerations would indicate the most prudent course of action to be that of providing each and every survivor of myocardial infarction with at least a screening interview to determine the extent of emotional distress and the potential for abnormal illness behaviors, and to offer a systematic program of psychological intervention where this is indicated by need. This implies the regular involvement of an individual designated to provide psychological intervention within the cardiological team. The final decision to provide psychological intervention or not is, of course, one that will be influenced by resources and facilities. Thus, a cardiological unit with adequate staff and space may opt to routinely advise its patients to become involved in a psychologically oriented program of rehabilitation just as it might routinely recommend a systematic process of exercise retraining. On the other hand, where resources are short, it may only be those with specifically identified psychological needs who can be offered the opportunity to participate in a program of psychological intervention. Thus, a single screening interview, with intervention given only on the basis of identified need, should be seen as the absolute minimum service that a cardiology unit should offer its patients.

The majority of studies evaluating the effects of psychological intervention following myocardial infarction have been conducted in groups. As is pointed out in Chapter 5, this has the twofold advantage of allowing for the more economical treatment of patients and of providing an appropriate environment in which concerns can be openly discussed and adaptive behaviors rehearsed. On the other hand, the acutely ill patient who remains in hospital may not be able to participate in group activities. For some patients, the potential for self-exposure arising out of involvement in a group may be sufficiently threatening to them to preclude their active participation. For these patients, individual intervention may be necessary; though for the latter group, it would seem wise to encourage their eventual assimilation into a group so that the benefits that come from this experience would not be entirely denied to them.

Recommendations regarding the stage of illness at which psychological intervention is offered vary between authorities. Gruen (1975) has advocated that psychological intervention should begin as early as possible certainly while the patient remains in the coronary-care unit. The work of Naismith and her colleagues (Naismith et al., 1979) suggests that, while intervention might start during the hospital phase, it is most effective if it is drawn out into the period of posthospital recovery. The majority of evaluated programs of psychological intervention have, however, been offered entirely in the posthospital phase of rehabilitation. Razin's (1982) review of the literature led him to conclude that the benefits to be gained from the early implementation of psychological intervention must be given very careful consideration in the decision as to when to commence this process. Once more, however, the decision may reduce to one of clinical convenience, where the capacity of the cardiological unit to schedule the commencement of psychological intervention into the process of medical management assumes greatest weight in the clinical decision. Psychological intervention must, of necessity, be interwoven into the whole fabric of management, where considerable emphasis may be paid to physical reconditioning. Nor can one ignore the possibility that, rather than involving a broadly based program of activity, psychological intervention may be focused on a specific problem behavior—for example, the need to eliminate smoking behavior or to enhance compliance with medical directions. This will, to a large extent, dictate the timing of psychological intervention and limit it to a period more related to medical management than to the patient's specific psychological needs.

Of course, generalization of behavior change to the natural environment is most likely to take place if psychological intervention itself occurs at least partly away from the hospital environment and in the patient's familiar premorbid social, personal, and occupational settings. Thus, while the lead set by Gruen (1975) and echoed by Razin (1982), that psychological intervention should commence as early as possible after myocardial infarction, presents a clearly sensible beginning, the extension of such intervention into the posthospital phase, as exemplified by the work of Naismith et al. (1979), would seem to offer the most broadly applicable, practical structure.

4. PATIENT ACCEPTANCE

For reasons largely related to the mobilization of denial, a considerable proportion (perhaps half) of patients surviving myocardial infarction are either reluctant to accept that they have, in fact, suffered a life-threatening illness or are eager to downplay its severity and personal significance when questioned (Byrne, Whyte, & Lance, 1978). Among those patients who do accept the reality of myocardial infarction, there is often a reluctance to accept that factors other than identified physical risks have contributed. It is not surprising, then, that among some groups of patients, at least, there is an unwillingness to accept that psychological intervention will be useful in the reduction of disability and discomfort and the prolongation of life (Langosch et al., 1982). As reported in the previous chapter, compliance rates with overall programs of psychological intervention following myocardial infarction range between around 70% and 85%; however, fewer patients demonstrate their compliance by attending all sessions of any given program. It might be inferred from this that programs of psychological intervention have a less-than-perfect acceptance among survivors of myocardial infarction. However, when one compares these data with attendance rates at programs solely emphasizing physical rehabilitation, with no reference to the patient's psychological state, one observes that compliance rates are of the same order, indicating that patient acceptance of protracted strategies of intervention represents a general difficulty rather than one specifically related to psychological intervention.

Some (for example, Gruen, 1975; Fielding, 1980) have, in their initial approaches to patients, deliberately avoided references to the terms "psychology" or "psychological." They emphasized, instead, their roles as members of a health-care team operating as part of the cardiological team's overall management strategy. Acceptance of psychological intervention was in these cases found to be somewhat higher than where more specific labels such as "group therapy" were attached to the service being offered (for example, Rahe et al., 1979). It may therefore be useful to adopt introductions de-emphasizing the psychological notion of intervention, lest it imply notions of instability and reduce the acceptability of the service. On the other hand, the clinician should signify an acceptance of the expression of emotional problems, fears, and concerns regarding disability and survival so that patients feel these issues may be freely discussed at a time of their choosing. In this respect, the approach outlined by Gruen (1975) has much to recommend it.

5.   ROLES AND RESPONSIBILITIES

Perhaps one of the most sensitive clinical issues in the psychological management of the cardiac patient has to do with roles, responsibilities, and territoriality. The physician has a long-standing and undeniably important role in the overall management of the cardiac patient, and may be unwilling to relinquish even the smallest part of this to a clinician not trained in physical medicine. This may, to some extent, be a phenomenon that is disappearing with time. Doehrman (1977) reported that 24 out of 36 programs involving a psychological component in the rehabilitation of cardiac patients were run by clinicians not specifically trained in clinical psychology or psychiatry. Primary involvement in these programs seemed to come from physicians and nursing staff. The recent advent of behavioral medicine and health psychology, however, with their emphasis on the pivotal role of the psychologically trained clinician in the routine management of medical patients, would seem to be removing barriers that have been in place for so long.

While behavioral medicine has been variously defined (Surwit et al., 1982), it emphasises a symbiotic approach to patient management whereby the medically trained physician and the clinical psychologist cooperate with and complement one another in order to provide the patient with the broadest and most appropriate basis of care. The procedures outlined in those chapters of the present book dealing with intervention have, by and large, been conceived of, developed, and evaluated by clinical psychologists. They can, of course, be used by providers of health care trained in other areas. There is, for example, an emerging tendency for the involvement of nurses in psychological intervention (Naismith et al., 1979), at least when they are under the supervision of a physician. Studies in North America have, however, been more inclined to use clinical psychologists or psychiatrists as those directly involved in the intervention process. From the points of view of time, convenience, training, and interest, there is much to recommend the psychologically trained clinician as the person specifically designated to undertake psychological intervention. This does not of necessity remove the management of the cardiac patient or the supervision of the overall management program from the physician, but provides one more member of the cardiac team to work in the patient's best interests. While these moves may initially be met with some resistance from those clinicians irrevocably wedded to technological medicine, the continued demonstration of benefits to be gained from psychological intervention, together with the continued involvement of clinical psychologists and others in the overall care of cardiac patients, should establish, over time, a permanent niche for the clinical psychologist in the cardiological service.

6. CONCLUSIONS

The past five years alone have seen the appearance of several complete volumes and many more research papers documenting, from an epidemiological perspective, the influence of psychological factors on cardiovascular disease and evaluating the effectiveness of psychological procedures designed to benefit the cardiac patient. As is the case with any new endeavor, blind alleys have been encountered; but along with these, many fruitful paths have been opened up, and the process of exploration continues. This exploration is consistently rewarded with encouraging findings. The continued accumulation of supportive evidence leaves little room for serious doubt now, either that aspects of personality and behavior contribute to the development of coronary heart disease, or that attention to the psychological needs of the survivor of myocardial infarction contributes in significant and important ways to the reduction of disability and the enhancement of survival.

This book has attempted to document the course of recovery and rehabilitation following myocardial infarction and to present the evidence relating to the determinants of that course. It has taken up the argument that therapeutic attention to the psychological and behavioral components of the complex process determining outcome can achieve significant gains for the cardiac patient, whether these be judged according to continued personal well-being or prolonged cardiovascular health. In this sense, it is evident that the management of the cardiac patient is, in some respects, as much a psychological concern as a medical one.

Scientific evidence is not, of course, the sole criterion by which a set of clinical procedures is adopted as standard practice. The entry of clinical psychologists and other psychologically trained clinicians into the sensitive environment of the coronary-care unit, the cardiac ward, and the coronary-rehabilitation clinic must take place with the understanding and acceptance of the medical team whose rightful job it is to protect the physiological integrity of the patient's cardiovascular system in a period when it is especially vulnerable. This entry will, therefore, be gained not only by persuasive scientific evidence regarding the merits of psychological intervention but also by the clinical psychologists' adoption and expression of an attitude of caring concern for the patient, a professionalism worthy of a responsible and ethical practitioner, and a recognition and understanding of the complex and delicate psychobiological situation within which the patient presently exists. If this can be achieved, the benefits will be evident both for the clinical psychologist and the physician; but most importantly, the benefits will be apparent for the patient and this, after all, must be the sole objective of any clinical endeavor.

References

Aberg, H., Hadstrand, H., & Lithell, H. (1980). Blood pressure control in a middle-aged male population. A 6–9 year follow-up with special reference to the problem of non-responders. *Acta Medica Scandinavica, 208,* 467–471.

Abernethy, J.D. (1976). The problem of non-compliance in long-term antihypertensive therapy. *Drugs, 11,* 86–90.

Adsett, C.A., & Bruhn, J.G. (1968). Short term group psychotherapy with post-myocardial infarction patients and their wives. *Canadian Medical Association Journal, 99,* 577–584.

Ahlmark, G., Ahlberg, G., Saetre, H., Haglund, I., & Korsgren, M. (1979). A controlled study of early discharge after uncomplicated myocardial infarction. *Acta Medica Scandinavica, 206,* 87–91.

Alderman, M.H., & Schoenbaum, E.E. (1975). Detecfion and treatment of hypertension at the work site. *New England Journal of Medicine, 293,* 65–68.

Anderson, J.R., & Waldron, I. (1983). Behavioral and content components of the structured interview assessment of the Type A behavior pattern in women. *Journal of Behavioral Medicine, 6,* 123–135.

Andrew, G.M., Oldridge, N.B., Parker, T.O., Cunningham, D.A., Rechnitzer, P.A., Jones, N.L., Buck, C., Kavanagh, T., Shephard, R.T., & Sutton, T.R. (1981). Reasons for dropout from exercise programs in post-coronary patients. *Medicine and Science Sport and Exercise, 13,* 164–168.

Andrews, G., MacMahon, S.W., Austin, A., & Byrne, D.G. (1982). Hypertension: Comparison of drug and non-drug treatments. *British Medical Journal, 283,* 1523–1532.

Ardlie, N., Glew, G., & Schwartz, C. (1966). Influence of catecholamines on nucleotide-induced platelet aggregation. *Nature, 212,* 415–417.

Armstrong, B.K., Mann, J.I., Adelstein, A.M., & Eskin, F. (1975). Commodity consumption and ischaemic heart disease mortality with special reference to dietary practices. *Journal of Chronic Diseases, 28,* 455–463.

Baile, W.F., & Engel, B.T. (1978). A behavioral strategy for promoting treatment compliance following myocardial infarction. *Psychosomatic Medicine, 40,* 413–419.

Baile, W.F., Brinker, J.A., Wachspress, J.D., & Engel, B.T. (1979). Signouts against medical advice from a coronary care unit. *Journal of Behavioral Medicine, 2,* 85–92.

Baili, I.R. (1979). Long-term effect of relaxation on blood pressure and anxiety levels of essential hypertensive males: A controlled study. *Psychosomatic Medicine, 41,* 637–646.

Bandura, A.A. (1978). Self-efficacy: Toward a unified theory of behavioral change. *Advances in Behavior Research and Therapy, 1,* 139–161.

Barefoot, J.C., Dahlstrom, W.G., & Williams, R.B. (1983). Hostility, CHD incidence and total mortality: A 25 year follow-up of 255 physicians. *Psychosomatic Medicine, 45,* 59–63.

Bass, C. (1984). Type A behavior in patients with chest pain: Test-retest reliability and psychometric correlates of Bortner scale. *Journal of Psychosomatic Research, 28,* 289–300.

Beck, T.A. (1967). *Depression: Clinical, experimental, and theoretical aspects.* London: Staple Press.

Becker, M.H., & Maiman, L.A. (1975). Sociobehavioral determinants of compliance with health and medical care recommendations. *Medical Care, 13,* 10–14.

Benson, H., Rosner, B.A., & Marzetta, B.R. (1973). Decreased systolic blood pressure in hypertensive subjects who practiced meditation. *Journal of Clinical Investigation, 52,* 8.

Benson, H., Rosner, B.A., & Marzetta, B.R. (1974a). Decreased blood pressure in pharmacologically treated hypertensive patients who regularly elicited the relaxation response. *Lancet, 1,* 289–291.

Benson, H., Rosner, B.A., & Marzetta, B.R. (1974b). Decreased blood pressure in borderline hypertensives who practiced meditation. *Journal of Chronic Diseases, 27,* 163–169.

Bernstein, D.A., & McAlister, A. (1976). The modification of smoking behavior: Progress and problems. *Addictive Behavior, 1,* 89–102.

Best, J.A., Owen, L.E., & Trentadue, L. (1978). Comparison of satiation and rapid smoking in self-managed smoking cessation. *Addictive Behavior, 3,* 71–78.

Bilodeau, C.B., & Hackett, T.P. (1971). Issues raised in a group setting by patients recovering from myocardial infarction. *American Journal of Psychiatry, 128,* 73–78.

Blanchard, E.B., Young, L.D., & Haynes, M.R. (1975). A simple feedback system for the treatment of elevated blood pressure. *Behavior Therapy, 6,* 241–245.

Blanchard, E.B., & Miller, S.T. (1977). Psychological treatment of cardiovascular disease. *Archives of General Psychiatry, 34,* 1402–1413.

Blittner, M., Goldberg, J., & Merbaum, M. (1978). Cognitive self-control factors in the reduction of smoking behavior. *Behavior Therapy, 2,* 553–561.

Blumenthal, J.A., Williams, R., Kong, Y., Schanberg, S.M., & Thompson, L.W. (1978). Type A behavior and angiographically documented coronary disease. *Circulation, 58,* 634–639.

Bortner, R.W. (1969). A short rating scale as a potential measure of Pattern A behavior. *Journal of Chronic Diseases, 22,* 87–91.

Brand, R.J. (1978). Coronary-prone behavior as an independent risk factor for coronary heart disease. In T.M. Dembroski, S.M. Weiss, J.L. Shields, Suzanne G. Haynes, M. Feinleib (Eds.), *Coronary-prone Behavior.* New York: Springer-Verlag.

Brand, R.J., Rosenman, R.H., Jenkins, C.D., Sholtz, R.I., & Zyzanski, S.J. (1978). Comparison of coronary heart disease prediction in the Western Collaborative Group Study using the structured interview and the Jenkins Activity Survey Assessments of the coronary-prone Type A behavior pattern. Cited in T.M. Dembroski et al. *Coronary Prone Behavior.* New York: Springer Verlag.

Braunwald, E., Ross, J., & Sonnenblick, E.H. (1976). Mechanisms of contraction of the normal failing heart. Boston: Little Brown.

Briggs, W. A., Lowenthal, D.T., Cirksena, W.J., Price, W.E., Gibson, T.P., & Flamenbaum, W. (1975). Propranolol in hypertensive dialysis patients: Efficacy and compliance. *Clinical Pharmacology and Therapeutics, 18,* 606–612.

Brown, J.S., & Rawlinson, M.E. (1977). Sex differences in sick role rejection and in work performance following cardiac surgery. *Journal of Health and Social Behavior, 18,* 276–292.

Bruce, E.H., Frederick, R., Bruce, R.A., & Fisher, L.D. (1976). Comparison of active participants and dropouts in Capri cardiopulmonary rehabilitation programs. *American Journal of Cardiology, 37,* 53–60.

Bruhn, J.G., Wolf, S., & Philips, B.U. (1971). *Journal of Psychosomatic Research, 15,* 305–313.

Burns, B.H. (1969). Chronic chest disease, personality and success in stopping cigarette smoking. *British Journal of Preventive and Social Medicine, 23,* 23–27.

Burt, A., Thornley, P., Illingsworth, D., White, P., Shaw, T.R., & Turner, R. (1974). Stopping smoking after myocardial infarction. *Lancet, 1,* 304–306.

Byrne, D.G. (1979). Anxiety as state and trait following survived myocardial infarction. *British Journal of Social and Clinical Psychology, 18,* 417–423.

Byrne, D.G. (1980). Attributed responsibility for life events of myocardial infarction. *Psychotherapy and Psychosomatics, 33,* 7–13.

Byrne, D.G. (1980). Effects of social context on psychological responses to survived myocardial infarction. *International Journal of Psychiatry in Medicine, 10,* 23–31.

Byrne, D.G. (1981). Type A behaviour, life events and myocardial infarction: Independent or related risk factors? *British Journal of Medical Psychology, 54,* 371–377.

Byrne, D.G. (1981). Sex differences in the reporting of symptoms of depression in the general population. *British Journal of Clinical Psychology, 20,* 83–92.

Byrne, D.G. (1982). Illness behaviour and psychosocial outcome after heart attack. *British Journal of Clinical Psychology, 21,* 145–146.

Byrne, D.G. (1982). Psychological responses to illness and outcome after survived myocardial infarction: A long term follow-up. *Journal of Psychosomatic Research, 26,* 105–112.

Byrne, D. G., & Rosenman, R.H. (1986). The Type A behavior pattern as a precursor to stressful life events: A confluence of coronary risks. *British Journal of Medical Psychology, 59,* 75–82.

Byrne, D.G., Rosenman, R.H., Schiller, E. & Chesney, M.A. (1985). Consistency and variation among instruments purporting to measure the Type A behavior pattern. *Psychosomatic Medicine, 47,* 242–261.

Byrne, D.G., & Whyte, H.M. (1978). Dimensions of illness behaviour in survivors of myocardial infarction. *Journal of Psychosomatic Research, 22,* 485–491.

Byrne, D.G., Whyte, H.M. (1979). Severity of illness and illness behaviour: A comparative study of coronary care patients. *Journal of Psychosomatic Research, 23,* 57–61.

Byrne, D.G., & Whyte, H.M. (1980). Life events and myocardial infarction revisited: The role of measures of individual impact. *Psychosomatic Medicine, 42,* 1–10.

Byrne, D.G., & Whyte, H.M. (1983). State and trait anxiety correlates of illness behaviour in survivors of myocardial infarction. *International Journal of Psychiatry in Medicine, 13,* 1–9.

Byrne, D.G., Whyte, H.M., & Lance, G.N. (1978). A typology of responses to illness in survivors of myocardial infarction. *International Journal of Psychiatry in Medicine, 9,* 135–145.

Byrne, D.G., Whyte, H.M., & Butler, K.L (1981). Illness behaviour and outcome following survived myocardial infarction: A prospective study. *Journal of Psychosomatic Research, 25,* 97–107.

Byrne, D.G., Rosenman, R.H., & Schiller, E. (1985). Patterns of dietary intake and serum lipids in a sample of employed, Australian males. Unpublished Manuscript, Department of Psychology, Australian National University.

Caffrey, B. (1968). Reliability and validity of behavioral measures in a study of coronary heart disease. *Journal of Chronic Diseases, 21,* 191–204.

Caffrey, B. (1978). Psychometric procedures applied to the assessment of the coronary-prone behavior pattern. In S.M. Weiss, J.L. Shields, S.G. Haynes, M. Feinlab (Eds.), *Coronary-Prone Behavior.* New York: Springer-Verlag.

Carmody, T.P., Senner, J.W., Malinow, M.R., & Matarazzo, J.D. (1980). Physical exercise rehabilitation: Long-term dropout rate in cardiac patients. *Journal of Behavioral Medicine, 3,* 163–168.

Carnahan, J.E., & Nugent, C.A. (1975). The effects of self-monitoring by patients on the control of hypertension. *American Journal of Medical Science, 269,* 69–73.

Caron, H.S., & Roth, H.P. (1968). Patients' cooperation with a medical regimen. *Journal of the American Medical Association, 203,* 922–926.

Case, R.B., Heller, S.S., & Shamai, E. (1983). Type A behavior and survival after myocardial infarction. *Circulation, 68, 29, Supplement 3.*

Cassem, N.H., & Hackett, T.P. (1971). Psychiatric consultation in a coronary unit. *Annals of Internal Medicine, 75,* 9–14.

Cassem, N.H., & Hackett, T.P. (1973). Psychological rehabilitation of myocardial infarction patients in the acute phase. *Heart and Lung, 2,* 382–388.

Caulfield, J.B. (1977). Anatomy of the cardiovascular system. In J.T. Willerson, C.A. Sanders (Eds.), *Clinical cardiology,* New York: Grune & Stratton.

Cautela, J.R. (1970). Treatment of smoking by covert sensitization. *Psychological Reports, 26,* 415–420.

Cay, E.L., Vetter, N., Philip, A.E., & Dugard, P. (1972). Psychological status during recovery from an acute heart attack. *Journal of Psychosomatic Research, 16,* 425–435.

Cay, E.L., Vetter, N., Philip, A.E., & Dugard, P. (1972). Psychological reactions to a coronary care unit. *Journal of Psychosomatic Research, 16,* 437–447.

Cay, E.L., Vetter, N.J., Philip, A.E., & Dugard, P. (1973). Return to work after a heart attack. *Journal of Psychosomatic Research, 17,* 231–243.

Cay, E.L., Philip, A.E., & Aitken, C.B. (1976). Psychological aspects of cardiac rehabilitation. In O. Hill (Ed.), *Modern trends in psychosomatic medicine.* London: Butterworth.

Chesney, M.A. (1978). Coronary-prone behavior and coronary heart disease: Intervention strategies. Unpublished Manuscript.

Chesney, M.A., Eagleston, J.R., & Rosenman, R. (1980). The Type A structured interview: A behavioral assessment in the rough. *Journal of Behavioral Assessment, 2,* 255–272.

Chesney, M.A., Eagleston, J.R., & Rosenman, R.H. (1981). Type A behavior: Assessment and intervention. In C.K. Prokop, L.A. Bradley (Eds.), *Medical Psychology,* New York: Academic Press.

Chesney, M.A., & Rosenman, R.H. (1980). Type A behavior in the work setting. In C.L. Cooper, R. Payne (Eds.), *Current concerns in occupational stress.* New York: John Wiley & Sons Ltd.,

Chesney, M.A., Black, G.W., Chadwick, J.H., & Rosenman, R.H. (1981). Psychological correlates of the Type A behavior pattern. *Journal of Behavioral Medicine, 4,* 217–229.

Christensen, D., Ford, M., Reading, J., & Castle, C.H. (1977). Sudden death in the late hospital phase of acute myocardial infarction. *Archives of Internal Medicine, 137,* 1675–1679.

Claiborn, W.L., Lewis, P., & Humble, S. (1972). Stimulus satiation and smoking: A revisit. *Journal of Clinical Psychology, 28,* 416–419.

Cohen, J.B. (1978). The influence of culture on coronary-prone behavior. In T.M. Dembroski, S.M. Weiss, J.L. Shields, Suzanne G. Haynes, M. Feinleib (Eds.), *Coronary-prone behavior.* New York: Springer-Verlag.

Cohen, J.B., Matthews, K.A., & Waldron, I. (1978). Section summary: Coronary-prone behavior, developmental and cultural considerations. In T.M. Dembroski, S.M. Weiss, J.L. Shields, S.G. Haynes, M. Feinleib (Eds.), *Coronary-prone behavior.* New York: Springer-Verlag.

Cohen, J.B., Syme, S.L., Jenkins, C.D., Kagan, A., & Zyzanski, S.J. (1975). The cultural context of Type A behavior and the risk of CHD. *American Journal of Epidemiology, 102,* 434.

Crain, R.B., & Missal, M.E. (1956). The industrial employee with myocardial infarction and his ability to return to work: Follow-up report. *New England Journal of Medicine, 56,* 2238–2244.

Crampton, R.S., Aldrich, R.F., Gascho, J.A., Miles, J.R., & Stillerman, R. (1975). Reduction of pre-hospital, ambulance and community coronary death rates by the community wide emergency cardiac care system. *American Journal of Medicine, 58,* 151–165.

Croog, S.H., Shapiro, D.S., & Levine, S. (1971). Denial among heart patients. *Psychosomatic medicine, 33,* 385–392.

Croog, S.H., & Levine, S. (1977). *The heart patient recovers.* New York: Human Sciences Press.

Croog, S.H., & Richards, N.P. (1977). Health beliefs and smoking patterns in heart patients and their wives: A longitudinal study. *American Journal of Public Health, 67,* 921–930.

Curtis, J. (1974). *The effects of educational intervention on the Type A behavior pattern.* Unpublished manuscript, University of Utah.

Danaher, B.G. (1978). Rapid smoking and self-control in the modification of smoking behavior. *Journal of Consulting and Clinical Psychology, 45,* 1068–1075.

Danaher, B.G. (1977). Research on rapid smoking: Interim summary and recommendations. *Addictive Behavior, 2,* 151–166.

Davidson, D.M., Winchester, M.A., Taylor, C.B., Alderman, E.A., & Ingels, N.B. (1979). Effects of relaxation therapy on cardiac performance and sympathetic activity in patients with organic heart disease. *Psychosomatic Medicine, 41,* 303–309.

Degré-Coustry, C., & Grevisse, M. (1982). Psychological problems in rehabilitation after myocardial infarction. *Advances in Cardiology, 29,* 126–131.

Dellipiani, A.W., Cay, E.L., Philip, A.E., Vetter, N.J., Colling, W.A., Donaldson, R.J., & McCormick, P. (1976). Anxiety after a heart attack. *British Heart Journal, 38,* 752–757.

Dembroski, T.M., Macdougall, J.M., & Shields, J.L. (1977). Physiologic reactions to social challenge in persons evidencing the Type A coronary-prone behavior pattern. *Journal of Human Stress, 3,* 2–9.

Dembroski, T.M., Macdougall, J.M., Shields, J.L., Petitto, J., & Lushene, R. (1978). Components of the Type A coronary-prone behavior pattern and cardiovascular responses to psychomotor performance challenge. *Journal of Behavioral Medicine, 1,* 159–176.

Dembroski, T.M., Weiss, S.M., Shields, J.L., Haynes, S.G., & Feinleib, M. (1978). *Coronary-prone behavior.* New York: Springer-Verlag.

Diederiks, J.P., van der Sluijs, H., Weeda, H.W., & Schobre, M.G. (1983). *Scandinavian Journal of Rehabilitation Medicine, 15*, 103–107.

Dimsdale, J.E., Hackett, T.P., Block, P.C., & Hutter, A.M. (1978). Emotional correlates of Type A behavior pattern. *Psychosomatic Medicine, 40*, 580–583.

Dimsdale, J.E., & Heid, J.A. (1982). Variability of plasma lipids in response to emotional arousal. *Psychosomatic Medicine, 44*, 413–430.

Doehrman, S.R. (1977). Psychosocial aspects of recovery from coronary heart disease: A review. *Social Science and Medicine, 11*, 199–218.

Dominian, J., & Dobson, M. (1969). Psychological attitudes to a coronary care unit. *British Medical Journal, 4*, 705–799.

Donovan, J.W. (1977). Randomized controlled trial of anti-smoking advice in pregnancy. *British Journal of Preventive and Social Medicine, 31*, 6–12.

Donovan, J.W., & Hodge, R.L. (1980). *Epidemiology of smoking and cardiovascular disease.* Canberra: National Heart Foundation of Australia.

Doyle, J.T., & Kannel, W.B. (1970). Coronary risk factors: 10 year findings in 7446 Americans. Paper presented to VI World Congress of Cardiology, London.

Dreyfuss, F., Dasberg, H. & Assael, M.I. (1969). The relationship of myocardial infarction to depressive illness. *Psychotherapy and Psychosomatics, 17*, 73–81.

Dunbar, J.M., Marshall, G.D., & Hovell, M.F. (1979). Behavioral strategies for improving compliance. In R.B. Haynes, D.W. Taylor, D.L. Sackett (Eds.), *Compliance in health care.* Baltimore: Johns Hopkins University Press.

Elder, S.T., & Eustis, N.K. (1975). Instrumental blood pressure conditioning in outpatient hypertensives. *Behavior Research and Therapy, 13*, 185–188.

Engel, B.T., Glasgow, M.S., & Gaardner, K.R. (1983). Behavioral treatment of high blood pressure: II. Follow-up results and treatment recommendations. *Psychosomatic Medicine, 45*, 23–29.

Epstein, L.H., & Collins, F.L. (1977). The measurement of situational influences on smoking. *Addictive Behavior, 2*, 47–53.

Espinosa de Restrepo, H. (1981). Four-year experience in a hypertension control program: Operation aspects. *Hypertension, 3*, 245–248.

Everitt, B.S. (1974). *Cluster analysis.* London: Heinemann Press.

Eysenck, H.H., & Fulker, D. (1982). The components of Type A behaviour and its genetic determinants. *Activitas Nervosa Superieur (Prague)*, Supplement 3, 111–125.

Ferner, J.D. (1980). *Successful time management.* New York: Wiley.

Fielding, R. (1980). A note on behavioural treatment in the rehabilitation of myocardial infarction patients. *British Journal of Social and Clinical Psychology, 19*, 157–161.

Finlayson, A., & McEwen, J. (1977). *Coronary heart disease and patterns of living.* London: Croom Helm.

Flaherty, J.T., & Weisfeldt, M.L. (1977). Myocardial infarction. In J.T. Willerson, C.A. Sanders (Eds.), *Clinical Cardiology,* New York: Grune & Stratton.

Fleming, J.S., & Braimbride, M.V. (1974). *Lecture Notes on Cardiology,* Oxford: Blackwell Scientific Publications.

Fletcher, S.W., Appel, F.A., & Bourgeois, M.A. (1975). Management of hypertension. Effect of improving patient compliance for follow-up care. *Journal of the American Medical Association, 233,* 242–244.

Foxx, R.M., & Brown, R.A. (1979). Nicotine fading and self-monitoring for cigarette abstinence or controlled smoking. *Journal of Applied Behavior Analysis, 12,* 111–125.

Francis, K.T. (1981). Perceptions of anxiety, hostility and depression in subjects exhibiting the coronary-prone behavior pattern. *Journal of Psychiatric Research, 16,* 183–190.

Frank, K.A., Keller, S.S., & Kornfeld, D.S. (1979). Psychological intervention in coronary heart disease. *General Hospital Psychiatry, 1,* 18–23.

Frankel, B.L., Patel, C., & Horwitz, D. (1977). Clinical ineffectiveness of a combination of psychophysiologic therapies. *Psychosomatic Medicine, 39,* 51–60.

Frankenhaeuser, M. (1976). Experimental approaches to the study of catecholamines and emotion. In L. Levi (Ed.), *Emotions: Their paramaters and measurement.* New York: Raven Press.

Frankenhaeuser, M. (1979). Psychoneuroendocrine approaches to the study of emotion as related to stress and coping. In H.E. Howe, R.A. Dienstbier (Eds.), *Nebraska symptosium on motivation.* Lincoln: University of Nebraska Press.

Frankenhaeuser, M., Lundberg, U., & Forsman, L. (1980a). Dissociation between sympathetic-adrenal and pituitary-adrenal responses to an achievement situation characterized by high controllability: Comparison between Type A and Type B males and females. *Biological Psychology, 10,* 79–91.

Frankenhaeuser, M., Lundberg, U., & Forsman, L. (1980b). Note on arousing Type A persons by depriving them of work. *Journal of Psychosomatic Research, 24,* 45–47.

Friedman, M. (1978). Modifying "Type A" behavior in heart attack patients. *Primary Cardiology,* 9–13.

Friedman, M. (1969). *Pathogenesis of coronary artery disease.* New York: McGraw-Hill.

Friedman, M., & Rosenman, R.H. (1959). Association of a specific overt behavior pattern with increases in blood cholesterol, blood clotting time, incidence of arcus senilis, and clinical coronary artery disease. *Journal of the American Medical Association, 169,* 1286–1296.

Friedman, M., & Rosenman, R.H. (1974). *Type A behavior and your heart.* New York: Knopf.

Friedman, M., Thoresen, C.E., Gill, J.J., Powell, L.H., Ulmer, D., Thompson, L., Price, V., Rabin, D., Breal, W.S., Dixon, T., Levy, R., & Bourg, E. (1984). Alteration of Type A behavior and reduction in cardiac recurrences in post myocardial infarction patients. *American Heart Journal, 108,* 237–248.

Froese, A.P., Cassem, N.H., Hackett, T.P., & Silverberg, E.L. (1975). Galvanic skin potential as a predictor of mental status, anxiety, depression and denial in acute coronary care patients. *Journal of Psychosomatic Research, 19,* 1–9.

Frumkin, K., Nathan, R.J., Prout, M.F., & Cohen, M.C. (1978). Non-pharmacologic control of essential hypertension in man: A critical review of the experimental literature. *Psychosomatic Medicine, 40,* 294–320.

Geersten, H.R., Ford, M., & Castle, C.H. (1976). The subjective aspects of coronary care. *Nursing Research, 25,* 211–215.

Gelman, M.L., & Nemati, C. (1981). A new method of blood pressure recording that may enhance patient compliance. *Journal of the American Medical Association, 246,* 368–370.

Gentry, W.D. (1978). Behavior modification of the coronary-prone behavior pattern. In T.M. Dembroski, S.M. Weiss, J.L. Shields, S.G. Haynes, M. Feinleib (Eds.), *Coronary-prone behavior.* New York: Springer-Verlag.

Gentry, W.D., Foster, S., & Haney, T. (1972). Denial as a determinant of anxiety and perceived health status in the coronary care unit. *Psychosomatic Medicine, 34*, 39–51.

Gentry, W.D., & Suinn, R.M. (1978). Section summary: Behavioral intervention. In T.M. Dembroski, S.M. Weiss, J.L. Shields, Suzanne G. Haynes, M. Feinleib (Eds.), *Coronary-prone behavior*. New York: Springer-Verlag.

Gerson, P., & Lanyon, R.I. (1972). Modification of smoking behavior with an aversion-desensitization procedure. *Journal of Consulting and Clinical Psychology, 38*, 399–402.

Gillum, R.F., Neutra, R.R., Stason, W.B., & Solomon, H.S. (1979). Determinants of dropout rate among hypertensive patients in an urban clinic. *Journal of Community Health, 5*, 94–100.

Glanz, K., Kirscht, J.P., & Rosenstock, I.M. (1981). Linking research and practice in patient education for hypertension: Patient responses to four educational interventions. *Medical Care, 19*, 141–152.

Glasgow, R.E. (1978). Effects of a self-control manual, rapid smoking and amount of therapist contact on smoking reduction. *Journal of Consulting and Clinical Psychology, 46*, 1430–1447.

Glass, D.C. (1977). *Behavior patterns, stress, and coronary disease*. Hillsdale, N.J.: Lawrence Erlbaum Associates.

Goldfried, M.R., & Merbaum, M. (1973). *Behavior change through self-control*. New York: Holt, Rinehart & Winston.

Goldberg, D.P. (1972). *The detection of psychiatric illness by questionnaire*. London: Oxford University Press.

Goldstein, I.B., Shapiro, D., Thananopavarn, C., & Sambhi, M.P. (1982). Comparison of drug and behavioral treatments of essential hypertension. *Health Psychology, 1*, 7–26.

Gordis, L. (1979). Conceptual and methodological problems in measuring patient compliance. In R.B. Haynes, D.W. Taylor, D.L. Sackett (Eds.), *Compliance in health care*. Baltimore, Johns Hopkins University Press.

Gotto, A.M., Miller, N.E., & Oliver, M.F. (Eds.). (1978). *High density lipoproteins and atherosclerosis*. Holland: Elsevier.

Green, E., & Green, A. *Beyond biofeedback*. New York: Dell Publishing Co.

Greenberg, I., & Altman, J.L. (1976). Modifying smoking behavior through stimulus control: A case study. *Journal of Behavior Therapy and Experimental Psychiatry, 7*, 97–99.

Groen, J.J. (1976). Psychosomatic aspects of ischaemic (coronary) heart disease. In O. Hill (Ed.), *Modern trends in psychosomatic medicine*. London: Butterworth.

Gruen, W. (1975). Effects of brief psychotherapy during the hospitalization period on the recovery process in heart attacks. *Journal of Consulting and Clinical Psychology, 43*, 223–232.

Hackett, G., & Horan, J.J. (1977). Behavioral control of cigarette smoking: A comprehensive programme. *Journal of Drug Education, 7*, 71–79.

Hackett, T.P. (1978). The use of groups in the rehabilitation of the post-coronary patient. *Advances in Cardiology, 24*, 127–135.

Hackett, T.P., Cassem, N.H., & Wishnie, H.A. (1968). The coronary care unit: An appraisal of psychological hazards. *New England Journal of Medicine, 279*, 1365.

Hackett, T.P., & Cassem, N.H. (1976). White and blue collar responses to heart attack. *Journal of Psychosomatic Research, 20*, 85–95.

Hahn, P., & Leisner, R. (1970). The influence of biographical anamnesis and group psychotherapy on post-myocardial patients. *Psychotherapy and Psychosomatics, 18,* 299.

Hall, R.G., Sachs, D.P.L. & Hall, S.M. (1970). Medical risks and therapeutic effectiveness of rapid smoking. *Behavior Therapy, 10,* 249–259.

Hall, S.M., Hall, D.M., & Gold, C.H. (1976). Hypertension detected in young black women by routine screening in a family clinic. *South African Medical Journal, 50,* 1198–1201.

Hallaq, J.H. (1976). The pledge as an instrument of behavioral change. *Journal of Social Psychology, 98,* 147–148.

Hammond, E.C., & Garfinkel, L. (1969). Coronary heart disease, stroke and aortic aneurism: Factors in the etiology. *Archives of Environmental Health, 19,* 167–182.

Haney, C.A. (1977). Illness behavior and psychosocial correlates of cancer. *Social Science and Medicine, 11,* 223–228.

Hartigan, J. (1976). *Clustering algorithms.* New York: Wiley.

Hauser, R. (1976). Rapid smoking as a technique of behavior modification: Caution in selection of subjects. *Journal of Consulting and Clinical Psychology, 42,* 625–626.

Hay, D.R., & Turbott, S. (1970). Changes in smoking habits in men under 65 years after myocardial infarction and coronary insufficiency. *British Heart Journal, 32,* 738–740.

Haynes, R.B. (1979). Introduction. In R.B. Haynes, D.W. Taylor, D.L. Sackett (Eds.), *Compliance in health care.* Baltimore: Johns Hopkins University Press.

Haynes, R.B., & Sackett, D.L., Gibson, E.S., Taylor, D.W., Hackett, B.C., Roberts, R.S., & Johnson, A.L. (1976). Improvement of medication compliance in uncontrolled hypertension. *Lancet, 1,* 1265–1268.

Haynes, R.B., Taylor, D.W., & Sackett, D.L. (1979). *Compliance in health care.* Baltimore: Johns Hopkins University Press.

Haynes, R.B., Taylor, D.W., Sackett, D.L., Gibson, E.S., Bernholz, C.D., & Mukherjee, J. (1980). Can simple clinical measurements detect patient noncompliance? *Hypertension, 2,* 757–764.

Haynes, S.G., Feinleib, M., & Kannel, W.B. (1980). The relationship of psychosocial factors to coronary heart disease in the Framingham Study: III. Eight year incidence of coronary heart disease. *American Journal of Epidemiology, 111,* 37–58.

Heller, R.F. (1979). Type A behavior and coronary heart disease. *British Medical Journal, 2,* 368.

Henderson, A.S. (1974). Care-eliciting behaviour in man. *Journal of Nervous and Mental Disease, 159,* 172–181.

Henderson, A.S., Byrne, D.G., & Duncan-Jones, P. (1981). *Neurosis and the social environment.* Sydney: Academic Press.

Herman, S., Blumenthal, J.A., Black, G.M., & Chesney, M.A. (1981). Self-ratings of Type A (coronary prone) adults: Do Type A's know they are Type A's. *Psychosomatic Medicine, 43,* 405–413.

Hodge, R.H., Jr., Lynch, S.S., Davison, J.P., Knight, J.G., Sinn, J.A., & Carey, R.M. (1979). Estimating compliance with diuretic therapy: Urinary hydrochlorothiazide-cocatinine ratios in normal subjects. *Hypertension, 1,* 537–542.

Horan, J.J., Hackett, G., Nicholas, W.C., Linberg, S.E., Stone, C.I., & Lukasi, H.C. (1977). Rapid smoking: A cautionary note. *Journal of Consulting and Clinical Psychology, 45,* 341–343.

Humphries, J.O. (1977). Survival after myocardial infarction: Prognosis and management. *Modern Concepts of Cardiovascular Disease, 46*, 51–56.

Ibrahim, M.A. (1976). The impact of intervention upon psychosocial functions of post-myocardial infarction patients. *South Carolina Medical Association Journal*, February Supplement, 23–26.

Ibrahim, M.A., Feldman, J.G., Sultz, H.A., Staiman, M.G., Young, L.J., & Dean, D. (1974). Management after myocardial infarction: A controlled trial of the effect of group psychotherapy. *International Journal of Psychiatry in Medicine, 5*, 253–268.

Inter-Society Commission for Heart Disease Resources. (1970). Report of the inter-society commission for heart disease resources: Primary prevention of the atherosclerotic diseases. *Circulation, 42*, A55–A95.

Irvine, J., Lyle, R.C., & Allon, R. (1982). Type A personality as psychopathology: Personality correlates and an abbreviated scoring system. *Journal of Psychosomatic Research, 26*, 183–189.

Israel, A.C., Raskin, P.A., & Pravder, M.D. (1979). The effects of self-monitoring of smoking and awareness of accuracy feedback upon a concurrent behavior. *Addictive Behavior, 4*, 199–203.

Jelinek, V.M., McDonald, I.G., Ryan, W.F., Ziffer, R.W., Clemens, A., & Gerloff, J. (1982). Assessment of cardiac risk 10 days after uncomplicated myocardial infarction. *British Medical Journal, 284*, 277–230.

Jenkins, C.D. (1978). A comparative review of the interview and questionnaire methods in the assessment of the coronary-prone behavior pattern. In T.M. Dembroski, S.M. Weiss, J.L. Shields, S.G. Haynes, M. Feinleib (Eds.), *Coronary-prone behavior*. New York: Springer.

Jenkins, C.D., Rosenman, R.H., & Friedman, M. (1967). Development of an objective psychological test for the determination of the coronary-prone behavior pattern in employed men. *Journal of Chronic Diseases, 20*, 371–379.

Jenkins, C.D., Rosenman, R.H., & Friedman, M. (1968). Replicability of rating the coronary prone behavior pattern. *British Journal of Preventive and Sociological Medicine, 22*, 16–22.

Jenkins, C.D., & Zyzanski, S.J. (1982). The Type A behaviour pattern is alive and well - when not dissected: A reply. *British Journal of Medical Psychology, 55*, 219–223.

Jenkins, C.D., Zyzanski, S.J., Rosenman, R.H., & Cleveland, G.L. (1971). Association of coronary-prone behavior scores with recurrence of coronary heart disease. *Journal of Chronic Diseases, 24*, 601–611.

Jenkins, D.C., Zyzanski, S.J., & Rosenman, R.H. (1979). *Jenkins activity survey manual (Form C)*. New York: The Psychological Corp.

Jenkins, C.D., Zyzanski, S.H., & Rosenman, R.H. (1976). Risk of new myocardial infarction in middle-aged men with manifest coronary heart disease. *Circulation, 53*, 342–347.

Jennings, J.R. (1984). Cardiovascular reactions and impatience in Type A and B college students. *Psychosomatic Medicine, 46*, 424–440.

Jennings, J.R., & Choi, S. (1981). Type A components and psychophysiological responses to an attention-demanding performance task. *Psychosomatic Medicine, 43*, 475–487.

Jennings, J.R., & Matthews, K.A. (1984). The impatience of youth: Phasic cardiovascular response in Type A and Type B elementary school-aged boys. *Psychosomatic Medicine, 46*, 498–511.

Jenni, M., & Wollersheim, J. (1979). Cognitive therapy, stress management training, and the Type A behavior pattern. *Cognitive Therapy and Research, 3,* 61–73.

Johnson, A. (1977). Sex differentials in coronary heart disease: explanatory role of primary risk factors. *Journal of Health and Social Behavior, 18,* 46–54.

Johnson, S.S. (1979). Health beliefs of hypertensive patients in a family medicine residency program. *Journal of Family Practice, 9,* 877–883.

Jorgensen, R.S., Houston, B.K., & Zuranski, R.M. (1981). Anxiety management training in the treatment of essential hypertension. *Behavior Research and Therapy, 19,* 467–474.

Kallio, V. (1982). Rehabilitation programmes as secondary prevention: A community approach. *Advances in Cardiology, 31,* 120–128.

Kallio, V., Hamalainen, H., Hakkila, J., & Luurila, O.J. (1979). Reduction in sudden deaths by a multi-factorial intervention programme after acute myocardial infarction. *Lancet, 2,* 1091–1094.

Kanfer, F.H. (1970). Self-monitoring: Methodological limitations and clinical applications. *Journal of Consulting and Clinical Psychology, 35,* 148–152.

Kannel, W.B., Dawber, T.R., & McNamara, P.M. (1966). Detection of the coronary-prone adult: The Framingham study. *Journal of the Iowa Medical Association, 56,* 26–34.

Kannel, W.B., McGee, D., & Gordon, T. (1976). A general cardiovascular profile: The Framingham study. *American Journal of Cardiology, 38,* 46–51.

Karstens, R., Kohle, K., & Ohlmeier, D. (1970). Multi-disciplinary approach for the assessment of psychodynamic factors in young adults with acute myocardial infarction. *Psychotherapy and Psychosomatics, 18,* 281–285.

Katz, N.W. (1979). Comparative efficacy of behavioral training, training plus relaxation and a sleep/trance hypnotic induction in increasing hypnotic susceptibility. *Journal of Consulting and Clinical Psychology, 47,* 119–127.

Keys, A. (1970). Coronary heart disease in seven countries. *Circulation, 41,* 1–211.

Klein, R.F., Kliner, V.A., Zipes, D.P., Troyer, W.G., & Wallace, A.G. (1968). Transfer from a coronary care unit. *Archives of Internal Medicine, 122,* 104–108.

Kornitzer, M., Kittel, F., De Backer, G., & Dramaix, M. (1981). The Belgian heart disease prevention project: Type A behavior pattern and the prevalence of coronary heart disease. *Psychosomatic Medicine, 43,* 133–145.

Kornitzer, M., De Backer, G., Dramaix, M., Kittel, F., Thilly, C., Graffar, K., & Vuylsteek, K. (1983). Belgian heart disease prevention project: Incidence and mortality results. *Lancet, 1,* 1066–1070.

Kottke, T.E., Young, D.T., & McCall, M.M. (1980). Effect of social class on recovery from myocardial infarction: A follow-up study of 197 consecutive patients discharged from hospital. *Minnesota Medicine, 63,* 590–597.

Kristt, D.A., & Engel, B.T. (1975). Learned control of blood pressure in patients with high blood pressure. *Circulation, 51,* 370–378.

Lakein, A. (1973). *How to get control of your time and your life.* New York: Signet.

Lamontagne, Y., & Gagnon, M.A. (1978). Thought stopping as a treatment for reducing cigarette smoking. *International Journal of Addictions, 13,* 297–305.

Lance, G.N., & Williams, W.T. (1975). REMUL: A new divisory polythetic classificatory programme. *Australian Computer Journal, 7,* 109–112.

Lando, H.A. (1977). Successful treatment of smokers with broad-spectrum behavioral approach. *Journal of Consulting and Clinical Psychology, 45,* 361–366.

Lando, H.A. (1978). Stimulus control, rapid smoking and contractual management in the maintenance of non-smoking behavior. *Behavior Therapy, 9,* 962–963.

Langosch, W., Seer, P., Brodner, G., Kallinke, D., Kulick, B., & Heim, F. (1982). Behavior therapy with coronary heart disease patients: Results of a comparative study. *Journal of Psychosomatic Research, 26,* 475–484.

Lazarus, R. (1966). *Psychological stress and the coping process.* New York: McGraw-Hill.

Lebovits, B.Z., Shekelle, R.B., & Ostfeld, A.M. (1967). Prospective and retrospective psychological studies of coronary heart disease. *Psychosomatic Medicine, 29,* 265–272.

Lee, R.L., & Ball, P.A. (1975). Some thoughts on the psychology of the coronary care unit patient. *American Journal of Nursing, 75,* 1498–1501.

Leeder, S.R., Dobson, A.J., Gibberd, R.W., & Flynn, S.J. (1983). Attack and case fatality rates for acute myocardial infarction in the Hunter region of New South Wales, Australia in 1979. *American Journal of Epidemiology, 118,* 42–51.

Levenberg, S.B., & Wagner, M.K. (1976). Smoking cessation: Long-term irrelevance of mode of treatment. *Journal of Behavior Therapy and Experimental Psychiatry, 7,* 93–95.

Levenkron, J.C., Cohen, J.D., Mueller, H.S., & Fisher, E.B. (1983). Modifying the Type A coronary-prone behavior pattern. *Journal of Consulting and Clinical Psychology, 51,* 192–204.

Levi, L. (Ed.). (1978). *Society, stress and disease, Volume 3. The productive and reproductive age - Male/female roles and relationships.* New York: Oxford University Press.

Levine, J., & Zigler, E. (1975). Denial and self-image in stroke, lung cancer and heart disease patients. *Journal of Consulting and Clinical Psychology, 43,* 751–757.

Lewittes, D.J., & Israel, A.C. (1975). Responsibility contracting for the maintenance of reduced smoking: A technique innovation. *Behavior Therapy, 6,* 696–698.

Ley, P. (1984). Satisfaction, compliance and communication. *British Journal of Clinical Psychology, 21,* 241–254.

Ley, P., & Morris, L.A. (1984). Psychological aspects of written information for patients. In S. Rachman (Ed.), *Contributions to Medical Psychology.* Vol. 3. Oxford: Pergamon Press.

Lechtenstein, E., & Keutzer, C.S. (1969). Experimental investigation of diverse techniques to modify smoking: A follow-up report. *Behavior Research and Therapy, 7,* 139–140.

Linde, B.J., & Janz, N.M. (1979). Effect of a teaching program on knowledge and compliance of cardiac patients. *Nursing Research, 28,* 282–286.

Lipowski, Z.J. (1970). Physical illness, the individual and the coping process. *International Journal of Psychiatry in Medicine, 1,* 21–100.

Lipowski, Z.J. (1975). Physical illness, the patient and his environment. In S. Arieti (Ed.), *American Handbook of Psychiatry.* New York: Basic Books.

Lipowski, Z.J., Lipsitt, D.R., & Whybrow, P.C. (1977). *Psychosomatic medicine: Current trends and clinical applications.* New York: Oxford University Press.

Lloyd, G.G., & Cawley, R.H. (1982). Psychiatric morbidity after myocardial infarction. *Quarterly Journal of Medicine, 51,* 33–42.

Lovell, R.R., Stephens, W.B., Thomson, L., & Ulman, R. (1976). The rate of initiation of treatment for hypertension in a community, 1971–1975. *Australian New Zealand Journal of Medicine, 6,* 398–401.

Lown, B., DeSilva, R.A., Reich, P., & Murawski, B.J. (1980). Psychophysiologic factors in sudden cardiac death. *American Journal of Psychiatry, 137,* 1325–1335.

Luborsky, L., Crits-Christoph, P., Brady, J.P., Kron, R.E., Weiss, T., Cohen, M., & Levy, L. (1982). Behavioral versus pharmacological treatments for essential hypertension: A needed comparison. *Psychosomatic Medicine, 44,* 203–213.

Lundberg, V., & Forsman, L. (1979). Adrenal-medullary and adrenal-cortical responses to understimulation and overstimulation: Comparison between Type A and Type B persons. *Biological Psychology, 9,* 79–89.

Lynch, J.J., Thomas, S.J., Mills, M.E., Malinow, K., & Katcher, A.H. (1974). The effects of human contact on cardiac arhythmia in coronary care patients. *Journal of Nervous and Mental Diseases, 158,* 83–99.

McAlister, A. (1975). Helping people quit smoking: Current progress. In A.J. Enelow, J.B. Henderson (Eds.), *Applying Behavioral Science to cardiovascular risk.* Washington: American Heart Association.

McAlister, A., Perry, C., & Maccoby, N. (1979). Adolescent smoking: Onset and prevention. *Pediatrics, 63,* 650–658.

McFall, R.M. (1970). Effects of self-monitoring on normal smoking behavior. *Journal of Consulting and Clinical Psychology, 35,* 135–142.

McFall, R.M. (1978). Smoking cessation research. *Journal of Consulting and Clinical Psychology, 46,* 703–712.

McGrath, M.J., & Hall, S.M. (1976). Self-management treatment of smoking behavior. *Addictive Behavior, 1,* 287–292.

Madsen, D., & McGuire, M.T. (1984). Whole blood serotonin and the Type A behavior pattern. *Psychosomatic Medicine, 46,* 546–548.

Mann, G.V. (1977). Diet-heart: End of an era. *New England Journal of Medicine, 297,* 644–650.

Manuck, S.B., & Garland, F.N. (1979). Coronary-prone behavior pattern, task incentive, and cardiovascular response. *Psychophysiology, 16,* 136–142.

Marmor, A., Sobel, B.E., & Roberts, R. (1981). Factors presaging early recurrent myocardial infarction (extension). *American Journal of Cardiology, 48,* 603–610.

Marmor, A., Geltman, E.M., Schechtman, K., Sobel, B.E., & Roberts, R. (1982). Recurrent myocardial infarction: Clinical predictors and prognostic implications. *Circulation, 66,* 415–421.

Marmot, M.G., & Syme, L. (1976). Acculturation and coronary heart disease in Japanese-Americans. *American Journal of Epidemiology, 104,* 225–247.

Marmot, M.G., Rose, G., Shipley, M., & Hamilton, P.J.S. (1978). Employment grade and coronary heart disease in British civil servants. *Journal of Epidemiology and Community Health, 32,* 244–249.

Martin, C.A., Thompson, D.L., Armstrong, B.K., Hobbs, M.S.T., & De Clerk, N. (1983). Long-term prognosis after recovery from myocardial infarction: A nine year follow-up of the Perth coronary register. *Circulation, 68,* 961–969.

Master, A.M., & Dack, S. (1940). Rehabilitation following acute coronary occlusion. *Journal of the American Medical Association, 115*, 828–832.

Masur, F.T. (1981). Adherence to health care regimens. In C.B. Prokop, L.A. Bradley (Eds.), *Medical psychology: Contributions to behavioral medicine*. New York: Academic Press.

Mather, H.G., Pearson, N.G., & Read, K.L.O. (1971). Acute myocardial infarction: Home and hospital treatment. *British Medical Journal, iii*, 334.

Matthews, K.A. (1978). Assessment and developmental antecedents of the coronary-prone behavior pattern in children. In T.M. Dembroski, S.M. Weiss, J.L. Shields, S.G. Haynes, M. Feinleib (Eds.), *Coronary-prone behavior*. New York: Springer-Verlag.

Matthews, K.A., & Krantz, D.S. (1976). Resemblances of twins and their parents in Pattern A behavior. *Psychosomatic Medicine, 38*, 140–144.

Matthews, K.A., Glass, D.C., & Richins, M. (1977). Behavioral interactions of mothers and children with the coronary-prone behavior pattern. In D.C. Glass (Ed.), *Behavior patterns, stress, and coronary disease*. Hillsdale, N.J.: Lawrence Erlbaum Associates.

Matthews, K.A., Glass, D.C., Rosenman, R.H., & Bortner, R.W. (1977). Competitive drive, pattern A and coronary heart disease: A further analysis of some data from the Western Collaborative Group Study. *Journal of Chronic Diseases, 30*, 489–498.

Matthews, K.A., Krantz, D.S., Dembroski, T.M., & McDougall, J.M. (1982). Unique and common variance in structured interview and Jenkins Activity Survey measures of the Type A behavior pattern. *Journal of Personality and Social Psychology, 42*, 303–313.

Matthews, K.A., Rosenman, R.H., Dembroski, T.M., Harris, E.L., & MacDougall, J.M. (1984). Familial resemblance in components of the Type A behavior pattern: A reanalysis of the California Type A twin study. *Psychosomatic Medicine, 46*, 512–522.

Mausner, J., Mausner, B., & Rial, W.Y. (1968). The influence of a physician on the smoking of his patients. *American Journal of Public Health, 58*, 46–53.

Mayou, R. (1979). The course and determinants of reactions to myocardial infarction. *British Journal of Psychiatry, 134*, 588–594.

Mayou, R. (1984). Prediction of emotional and social outcome after a heart attack. *Journal of Psychosomatic Research, 28*, 17–25.

Mayou, R., Williamson, B., & Foster, A. (1978a). Outcome two months after a myocardial infarction. *Journal of Psychosomatic Research, 22*, 447–453.

Mayou, R., Foster, A., & Williamson, B. (1978b). Psychosocial adjustment in patients one year after myocardial infarction. *Journal of Psychosomatic Research, 22*, 447–453.

Mayou, R., MacMahon, D., Sleight, P., & Florencio, M.J. (1981). Early rehabilitation after myocardial infarction. *Lancet, 2*, 1399–1402.

Mechanic, D. (1966). Response factors in illness: The study of illness behavior. *Social Psychiatry, 1*, 11–20.

Meichenbaum, D. (1977). *Cognitive behavior modification*. London: Plenum Press.

Mettlin, C. (1976). Occupational careers and the prevention of coronary-prone behavior. *Social Science and Medicine, 10*, 367–372.

Meyer, A.J., & Henderson, H.B. (1974). Multiple risk factor reduction in the prevention of cardiovascular disease. *Preventive Medicine, 3*, 225–236.

Miller, N.E. (1975). Applicaions of learning and biofeedback to psychiatry and medicine. In A.M.

Freedman, H.I. Kaplan, B.J. Sadock (Eds.), *Comprehensive textbook of psychiatry II*. Baltimore: Williams and Wilkins.

Mischel, W. (1976). *Introduction to personality*. New York: Holt, Rinehart & Winston.

Mone, L.C. (1970). Short-term group psychotherapy with post cardiac patients. *International Journal of Group Psychotherapy, 20*, 99–108.

Morganstern, K.P., & Ratliff, R.G. (1969). Systematic desensitization as a technique for treating smoking behavior: A preliminary report. *Behavior Research and Therapy, 7*, 397–398.

Morris, J.W. (1959). Occupation and coronary heart disease. *Archives of Internal Medicine, 104*, 903–907.

Moses, L., Daniels, G.E., & Nickerson, J.L. (1956). Psychogenic factors in essential hypertension. *Psychosomatic Medicine, 18*, 471–485.

Mulcahy, R. (1976). The rehabilitation of patients with coronary heart disease: A clinician's view. In U. Stocksmeier (Ed.), *Psychological approach to the rehabilitation of coronary patients*. Berlin: Springer.

Multiple risk factor intervention trial research group. Multiple risk factor intervention trial: Risk factor changes and mortality results. *Journal of the American Medical Association, 248*, 1465–1477.

Mushlin, A.I., & Appl, F.A. (1977). Diagnosing patient non-compliance. *Archives of Internal Medicine, 137*, 318–321.

Myrtek, M., & Greenlee, M.W. (1984). Psychophysiology of Type A behavior pattern: A critical analysis. *Journal of Psychomatic Research, 28*, 455–466.

Nagle, R., Gangola, R., & Picton-Robinson, I. (1971). Factors influencing return to work after an MI. *Lancet, 2*, 454–455.

Naismith, L.D., Robinson, J.F., Shaw, G.B., & MacIntyre, M.M.J. (1979). Psychological rehabilitation after myocardial infarction. *British Medical Journal, 1*, 439–442.

National Heart and Lung Institute. (1971). *Atherosclerosis*. DHEW Publication No. (NIH) 72–137.

Nelson, E.C., Stason, W.B., Neutra, R.R., Solomon, H.S., & McArdle, P.J. (1978). Impact of patient perceptions on compliance with treatment for hypertension. *Medical Care, 16*, 893–906.

Nelson, S.K. (1977). Behavioral control of smoking with combined procedures. *Psychological Reports, 40*, 191–196.

Nessman, D.G., Carnahan, J.E., & Nugent, C.A. (1980). Increasing compliance. Patient-operated hypertension groups. *Archives Internal Medicine, 140*, 1427–1430.

Nichols, A.B., Ravenscroft, C., Lamphiear, D.E., & Ostrander, L.D. (1976). Independence of serum lipid levels and dietary habits. *Journal of the American Medical Association, 236*, 1948–1953.

Norris, D.E., Caughey, D.E., Deeming, L.W., Mercer, C.J., & Scott, P.J. (1970). Coronary prognostic index for predicting survival after recovery from acute myocardial infarction. *Lancet, ii*, 485–488.

Novaco, R.W. (1975). *Anger control*. Lexington, Massachusetts: Heath.

Ohlmeier, D., Karstens, R., & Kohle, K. (1973). Psychoanalytic group interview and short-term psychotherapy with post-myocardial infarction patients. *Psychiatric Clinics, 6*, 240–249.

Oldenburg, B., & Perkins, R. (1984). Psychological intervention in myocardial infarction. Unpublished Manuscript. Department of Psychiatry, Prince Henry Hospital.

Oldridge, N.B., Donner, A.P., Buck, C.W., Jones, N.L., Andrew, G.M., Parker, J.O., Cunningham, D.A., Kavanagh, T., Rechnitzer, P.A., & Sutton, J.R. (1983). Predictors of dropout from cardiac exercise rehabilitation: Ontario exercise-heart collaborative study. *American Journal of Cardiology, 51,* 70–74.

Ohn, H.S., & Hackett, T.P. (1964). The denial of chest pain in 32 patients with acute myocardial infarction. *Journal of the American Medical Association, 190,* 977–981.

Orleans, C.T., Shipley, R.H., Williams, C., & Haac, L.A. (1981). Behavioral approaches to smoking cessation: II. Topical bibliography 1969–1979. *Journal of Behavior Therapy and Experimental Psychiatry, 12,* 131–144.

Osler, W. (1892). *The principles and practice of medicine.* Edinburgh: Young, J. Reutland.

Ostfeld, A.M., Lebovits, B.Z., & Shekelle, R.B. (1964). A prospective study of the relationship between personality and coronary heart disease. *Journal of Chronic Diseases, 17,* 265–276.

Parsons, T. (1951). *The social system.* Glencoe: Free Press.

Patel, C.H. (1975). Twelve month follow-up of yoga and biofeedback in the management of hypertension. *Lancet, 1,* 62–67.

Patel, C., Marmot, M.G., & Terry, D.J. (1981). Controlled trial of biofeedback-aided behavioural methods in reducing mild hypertension. *British Medical Journal, 282,* 2005–2008.

Pechacek, T.F., & McAlister, A.L. (1980). Strategies for the modification of smoking behavior: Treatment and prevention. In J.M. Ferguson, C.B. Taylor (Eds.), *The comprehensive handbook of behavioral medicine, Vol. 3.* New York: Spectrum Publications.

Peel, A.A.F., Semple, T., Wang, I., Lancaster, W.M., & Dall, J.L.G. (1960). A coronary prognostic index for grading the severity of infarction. *British Heart Journal, 24,* 743–760.

Peitzman, S.J., Bodison, W., & Ellis, I. (1982). Care of elderly patients in a special hypertension clinic. *Journal of American Geriatric Society, 30,* 2–5.

Pell, S., & D'Alonzo, C.A. (1963). Acute myocardial infarction in a large industrial population: Report of a 6 year study of 1,356 cases. *Journal of the American Medical Association, 185,* 831–838.

Philip, A.E., Cay, E.L., Vetter, N.J., & Stuckey, N.A. (1979). Personal traits and the physical, psychiatric and social state of patients one year after a myocardial infarction. *International Journal of Reabilitation Research, 2,* 479–487.

Philip, A.E., Cay, E.L., Stuckey, N.A., & Vetter, N.J. (1981). Multiple predictors and multiple outcomes after myocardial infarction. *Journal of Psychosomatic Research, 25,* 137–141.

Phillips, D.L., & Segal, B.E. (1969). Sexual status and psychiatric symptoms. *American Sociological Review, 34,* 58–72.

Pilowsky, I. (1967). Dimensions of hypochondriasis. *British Journal of Psychiatry, 113,* 89–93.

Pilowsky, I. (1969). Abnormal illness behaviour. *British Journal of Medical Psychology, 42,* 347–351.

Pilowsky, I., & Spence, N.D. (1975). Patterns of illness behaviour in patients with intractable pain. *Journal of Psychosomatic Research, 19,* 279–287.

Pincherle, G., & Wright, H.B. (1970). Doctor variation in reducing cigarette consumption. *The Practitioner, 205,* 209–213.

Pittner, M.S., & Houston, B.K. (1980). Response to stress, cognitive coping strategies, and the Type A behavior pattern. *Journal of Personality and Social Psychology, 39*, 147–157.

Pole, D.J., McCall, M.G., Reader, R., & Woodings, T. (1977). Incidence and mortality of acute myocardial infarction in Perth, Western Australia. *Journal of Chronic Diseases, 30*, 19–27.

Pollack, A.A., Weber, M.A., & Case, D.B. (1977). Limitations of transcendental meditation in the treatment of essential hypertension. *Lancet, 1*, 71–73.

Pooling Project Research Group. Relationship of blood pressure, serum cholesterol, smoking habit, relative weight, and ECG abnormalities to incidence of major coronary events: Final report of the pooling project. *Journal of Chronic Diseases, 31*, 201–306.

Powell, L.H., Friedman, M., Thoresen, C.E., Gill, J.J., & Ulmer, D.K. (1984). Can the Type A behavior pattern be altered after myocardial infarction? A second year report from the recurrent coronary prevention project. *Psychosomatic Medicine, 26*, 293–313.

Pozen, M.W., Stechmiller, J.A., Harris, W., Smith, S., Fried, D.D., & Voigt, G.C. (1977). A nurse rehabilitator's impact on patients with myocardial infarction. *Medical Care, 15*, 830–837.

Prince, R., & Miranda, L. (1977). Monitoring life stress to prevent recurrence of coronary heart disease episodes: Report of a feasibility study. *Canadian Psychiatric Association Journal, 22*, 161–169.

Pritchard, M. (1977). Further studies of illness behaviour in long-term haemodialysis. *Journal of Psychosomatic Research, 21*, 41–48.

Rahe, R.H., O'Neil, T., Hagan, A., & Arthur, R.J. (1975). Brief group therapy following myocardial infarction: Eighteen month follow-up of a controlled trial. *International Journal of Psychiatry in Medicine, 6*, 349–358.

Rahe, R.H., Ward, H.W., & Hayes, V. (1979). Brief group therapy in myocardial infarction rehabilitation: Three to four year follow-up of a controlled trial. *Psychosomatic Medicine, 41*, 229–242.

Razin, A.M. (1982). Psychosocial intervention in coronary artery disease: A review. *Psychosomatic Medicine, 44*, 363–387.

Reiser, M.F., Brust, A.A., & Ferris, E.B. (1951). Life situations, emotions and the course of patients with arterial hypertension. *Psychosomatic Medicine, 13*, 133–139.

Remmell, P.S., Gorder, D.D., Hall, Y., & Tillotson, J.L. (1980). Assessing dietary adherence in the multiple risk factor. *Journal of American Diet Association, 76*, 351–356.

Resnick, J. (1968). The control of smoking behavior by stimulus satiation. *Behavior Research and Therapy, 6*, 113–114.

Richards, C.S., & Perri, M.G. (1978). Do self-control treatments last?: An evaluation of behavioral problem solving and faded counsellor contact as treatment maintenance strategies. *Journal of Counseling Psychology, 25*, 376–383.

Rimm, D.C., & Masters, J.C. (1979). *Behavior therapy: Techniques and empirical findings, 2nd Edition.* New York: Academic Press.

Rose, G. (1975). The contribution of intensive coronary care. *British Journal of Preventive and Social Medicine, 29*, 147–150.

Rose, G., & Hamilton, P.J.S. (1978). A randomised controlled trial of the effect on middle-aged men of advice to stop smoking. *Journal of Epidemiology and Community Health, 32*, 275–281.

Rose, G., Tunstall-Pedoe, H.D., & Heller R.F. (1983). U.K. heart disease prevention project: Incidence and mortality results. *Lancet, i,* 1062–1065.

Rosen, J.L., & Bibring, G.L. (1966). Psychological reactions of hospitalized male patients to a heart attack. *Psychosomatic Medicine, 28,* 808–821.

Rosenman, R.H. (1981). *Psychosomatic risk factors and coronary heart disease: Indications for specific preventive therapy.* Bern, Stuttgart, Vienna: Hans Huber Publishers.

Rosenman, R.H. (1978). The interview method of assessment of the coronary-prone behavior pattern. In T.M. Dembroski, S.M. Weiss, J.L. Shields, S.G. Haynes, M. Feinleib (Eds.), *Coronary-prone behavior.* New York: Springer-Verlag.

Rosenman, R.H., & Chesney, M.A. (1980). The relationship of Type A behavior pattern to coronary heart disease. *Activitas Nervosa Superior, 22,* 1–45.

Rosenman, R.H., & Friedman, M. (1977). Modifying Type A behavior pattern. *Journal of Psychosomatic Research, 21,* 323–331.

Rosenman, R.H., Friedman, M. & Straus, R. (1964). A predictive study of coronary heart disease: The Western Collaborative Group Study. *Journal of the American Medical Association, 189,* 15–22.

Rosenman, R.H., Rahe, R.H., Borhani, N.O., & Feinleib, M. (1976). Heritability of personality and behavior. *Acta Geneticae Medicae et Gemellologiae, 25,* 221–224.

Rosenman, R.H., Friedman, M., & Jenkins, C.D. (1967). Recurring and fatal myocardial infarction in the Western Collaborative Group Study. *American Journal of Cardiology, 19,* 771–789.

Rosenman, R.H., Brand, R.J., Jenkins, C.D., Friedman, M., Straus, R., & Wurm, M. (1975). Coronary heart disease in the Western Collaborative Group Study. *Journal of the American Medical Association, 233,* 872–877.

Roskies, E., Kearney, H., Spevack, M., Surkis, A., Cohen, C., & Gilman, S. (1979). Generalizability and durability of treatment effects in an intervention program for coronary-prone (Type A)managers. *Journal of Behavioral Medicine, 2,* 195–207.

Roskies, F., Spevack, M., Surkis, A., Cohen, C., & Gilman, S. (1978). Changing the coronary-prone (Type A) behavior pattern in a non-clinical population. *Journal of Behavioral Medicine, 1,* 201–216.

Royal College of Physicians. (1975). Report of a joint working party: Cardiac rehabilitation. *Journal of the Royal College of Physicians of London, 9,* 281–346.

Ruberman, W., Weinblatt, E., Goldberg, J.D., & Chaudhary, B.S. (1983). Education, psychosocial stress and sudden cardiac death. *Journal of Chronic Diseases, 36,* 151–160.

Ruberman, W., Weinblatt, E., Goldberg, J.D., & Chaudhary, B.S. (1984). Psychosocial influences on mortality after myocardial infarction. *New England Journal of Medicine, 311,* 552–559.

Rudd, P., Tul, V., Brown, K., Davidson, S.M., & Bostwick, G.J. (1979). Hypertension continuation adherence: Natural history and role as an indicator condition. *Archives of Internal Medicine, 139,* 545–549.

Russell, M.A.H., Armstrong, E., & Patel, U.A. (1976). Temporal contiguity in electric aversion therapy for cigarette smoking. *Behavior Research and Therapy, 14,* 103–123.

Russell, M.A.H., Wilson, C., Taylor, C., & Baker, C.D. (1979). Effects of general practitioner's advice against smoking. *British Medical Journal, 10,* 231–235.

Sackett, D.L., Haynes, R.B., Gibson, E.S., Hackett, B.C., Taylor, D.W., Roberts, R.S., & Johnson, A.L. (1975). Randomised clinical trial of strategies for improving medication compliance in primary hypertension. *Lancet, 1,* 1205–1207.

Sackett, D.L.. & Snow, J.C. (1979). The magnitude of compliance and noncompliance. In R.B. Haynes, D.W. Taylor, D.L. Sackett (Eds.), *Compliance in health care.* Baltimore: Johns Hopkins University Press.

Salonen, J.T., & Puska, P. (1980). A community programme for rehabilitation and secondary prevention for patients with acute myocardial infarction as part of a comprehensive community programme for control of cardiovascular diseases. *Scandinavian Journal of Rehabilitation Medicine, 12,* 33–42.

Schachter, S. (1978). Pharmacological and psychological determinants of smoking. *Annals of Internal Medicine, 88,* 108–114.

Schachter, S. (1982). Recidivism and self-cure of smoking and obesity. *American Psychologist, 37,* 436–444.

Schaefer, E.J., Eisenberg, S., & Levy, R.I. (1978). Lipoprotein, apoprotein metabolism. *Journal of Lipid Research, 19,* 667–687.

Scherwitz, L., Berton, K., & Leventhal, H. (1978). Type A behavior, self-involvement and cardiovascular response. *Psychosomatic Medicine, 40,* 593–609.

Schmahl, D.P., Lichtenstein, E., & Harris, D.E. (1972). Successful treatment of habitual smokers with warm, smoky air and rapid smoking. *Journal of Consulting and Clinical Psychology, 38,* 105–111.

Schwartz, G.E., & Beatty, J. (1977). *Biofeedback: Theory and research.* New York: Academic Press.

Schwartz, G.E., & Shapiro, D. (1973). Biofeedback and essential hypertension: Current findings and theoretical concerns. In L. Birk (Ed.), *Biofeedback; Behavioral medicine.* New York: Grune & Stratton.

Seer, P. (1979). Psychological control of essential hypertension: Review of the literature and methodological critique. *Psychological Bulletin, 86,* 1015–1043.

Segers, M.J., & Mertens, C. (1975). Relationship between anxiety, depression, self-ratings and CHD risk factors among obese, normal and lean individuals. *Journal of Psychosomatic Research, 20,* 25–35.

Segers, M.J., & Mertens, C. (1977a). Personality aspects of CHD related behavior. *Journal of Psychosomatic Research, 21,* 79–85.

Segers, M.J., & Mertens, C. (1977b). Preventive behavior and awareness of myocardial infarction: A factorial definition of anxiety. *Journal of Psychosomatic Research, 21,* 213–223.

Seligman, M.E.P. (1975). *Helplessness. On depression, development and death.* San Francisco: Freeman.

Shapiro, D., Schwartz, G.E., Turksy, B., & Schnidman, S.R. (1971). Smoking on cue: A behavioral approach to smoking reduction. *Journal of Health and Social Behavior, 12,* 108–113.

Shapiro, D., Mainardi, J.A., & Surwit, R.S. (1977). Biofeedback and self-regulation in essential hypertension. In G.E. Schwartz, J. Beatty (Eds.), *Biofeedback: Theory and research.* New York: Academic Press.

Shapiro, D., & Surwit, R.S. (1979). Biofeedback. In O.F. Pomerlean, J.P. Brady (Eds.), Behavioral medicine: *Theory and practice.* Baltimore: Williams and Wilkins.

Shapiro, D., & Goldstein, I.B. (1983). Behavioral patterns as they relate to hypertension. In J. Rosenthal (Ed.), *Clinical pathophysiology of arterial hypertension*. New York: Springer.

Shapiro, S., Weinblatt, E., Frank, C.W., & Sager, R.V. (1969). Incidence of coronary heart disease in a population insured for medical care. *American Journal of Public Health, 59*, Supp. 6, 1–101.

Shekelle, R.B., Shryock, A.M., Paul, O., Lepper, M., Stamler, J., Liu, S., & Raynor, W.J. (1981). Diet, serum cholesterol and death from coronary heart disease. *New England Journal of Medicine, 304*, 65–70.

Shekelle, R.B., Gayle, M., Ostfeld, A.M., & Paul, O. (1983). Hostility, risk of coronary heart disease and mortality. *Psychosomatic Medicine, 45*, 109–114.

Silas, J.H., Tucker, G.T., & Smith, A.J. (1980). Drug resistance, inappropriate dosing and non-compliance in hypertensive patients. *British Journal of Clinical Pharmacology, 9*, 427–430.

Smith, T.W. (1984). Type A behavior, anger and neuroticism: The discriminant validity of self-reports in a patient sample. *British Journal of Clinical Psychology, 23*, 147–148.

Smith, T.W., Follick, M.J., & Korr, K.S. (1984). Anger, neuroticism, Type A behaviour and the experience of angina. *British Journal of Medical Psychology, 57*, 249–252.

Soloff, P.H. (1978). Denial and rehabilitation of the post-infarction patient. *International Journal of Psychiatry in Medicine, 8*, 125–132.

Soloff, P.H. (1979). Medically and surgically treated coronary patients in cardiovascular rehabilitation. *International Journal of Psychiatry in Medicine, 9*, 93–106.

Soloff, P.H. (1980). Effects of denial on mood, compliance, and quality of functioning after cardiovascular rehabilitation. *General Hospital Psychiatry, 2*, 134–140.

Southam, M.A., Agras, W.S., Taylor, C.B., & Kraemer, H.C. (1982). Relaxation training: Blood pressure lowering during the working day. *Archives of General Psychiatry, 39*, 715–717.

Speilberger, C.D. (1972). *Anxiety: Current trends in theory and research*. New York: Academic Press.

Spring, F.L., Sipich, J.F., Trimble, R.W., & Goeckner, D.J. (1978). Effects of contingency and non-contingency contracts in the context of a self-control oriented smoking modification program. *Behavior Therapy, 9*, 967–968.

Stamler, J. (1974). The prevention of coronary heart disease. In E. Braunwald (Ed.), *The myocardium: Failure and infarction*. New York: H.B. Publishing.

Stamler,R., Stamler, J., Civincelli, J., Pritchard, D., Gosch, F.C., Ticho, S., Restivo, B., & Fine, D. (1975). Adherence and blood-pressure response to hypertension treatment. *Lancet, 2*, 1227–1230.

Steffy, R.A., Meichenbaum, D., & Best, J.A. (1970). Aversive and cognitive factors in the modification of smoking behavior. *Behavior Research and Therapy, 8*, 115–125.

Stein, E.H., Murdaugh, J., & MacLeod, J.A. (1969). Brief psychotherapy for psychiatric reactions to physical illness. *American Journal of Psychiatry, 8*, 1040–1047.

Steptoe, A. (1981). *Psychological factors in cardiovascular disorders*. London: Academic Press.

Steptoe, A., & Ross, A. (1981). Psychophysiological reactivity and the prediction of cardiovascular disorders. *Journal of Psychosomatic Research, 25*, 23–31.

Stern, M.J., & Cleary, P. (1981). National exercise and heart disease project: Psychosocial changes observed during a low-level exercise programme. *Archives of Internal Medicine, 141*, 1463–1467.

Stern, M.J., & Cleary, P. (1982). The national exercise and heart disease project: Long-term psychosocial outcome. *Archives of Internal Medicine, 142,* 1093–1097.

Stone, G.C. (1979). Patient compliance and the role of the expert. *Jounal of Social Issues, 35,* 34–59.

Stone, R.A., & DeLeo, J. (1976). Psychotherapeutic control of hypertension. *New England Journal of Medicine, 294,* 80–84.

Suinn, R.M. (1978). The coronary-prone behavior pattern: A behavioral approach to intervention. In T.M. Dembroski, S.W. Weiss, J.L. Shields, S.G. Haynes, M. Feinleib (Eds.), *Coronary-prone behavior.* New York: Springer-Verlag.

Suinn, R.M. (1980). Pattern A behaviors and heart disease: Intervention approaches. In J.M. Ferguson & C.B. Taylor (Eds.), *Behavioral Medicine.* Lancaster: MTP Press.

Suinn, R.M. (1976). Anxiety management training to control general anxiety. In J. Krumboltz & C. Thoresen (Eds.), *Counseling Methods.* New York: Holt.

Suinn, R.M. (1972). Behavior rehearsal training for ski racers. Brief report. *Behavior Therapy, 3,* 519.

Suinn, R.M. (1975). The cardiac stress management program for Type A patients. *Cardiac Rehabilitation, 5(4).*

Suinn, R.M., & Bloom, L.J. (1978). Anxiety management training for Type A persons. *Journal of Behavioral Medicine, 1,* 25–35.

Suinn, R.M., & Richardson, F. (1971). Anxiety management training: A nonspecific behavior therapy program for anxiety control. *Behavior Therapy, 4,* 498.

Surwit, T.S., Shapiro, D., & Good, M.I. (1978). Comparison of cardiovascular biofeedback, neuromuscular biofeedback and meditation in the treatment of borderline essential hypertension. *Journal of Consulting and Clinical Psychology, 46,* 252–263.

Surwit, R.S., Williams, R.B., & Shapiro, D. (1982). *Behavioral approaches to cardiovascular disease.* New York: Academic Press.

Takala, J., Niemella, N., Rosti, J., & Sievers, K. (1979). Improving compliance with therapeutic regimens in hypertensive patients in a community health center. *Circulation, 59,* 540–543.

Takeuchi, M. (1983). In-hospital rehabilitation at the recovery phase after acute myocardial infarction. *Japanese Circulation Journal, 47,* 744–751.

Taylor, C.B., Farquhar, J.W., Nelson, E., & Agras, W.S. (1977). Relaxation therapy and high blood pressure. *Archives of General Psychiatry, 34,* 339–342.

Thockloth, R.M., Ho, S.C., Wright, H., & Seldon, W.A. (1973). Is cardiac rehabilitation really necessary? *Medical Journal of Australia, 2,* 669–674.

Thompson, E.L. (1978). Smoking education programs 1960–1976. *American Journal of Public Health, 68,* 250–257.

Thoresen, C.E., & Öhman, A. (1985). The Type A behavior pattern: A person-environment interaction perspective. In D. Magnusson, A. Öhman (Eds.), *Psychopathology: An interaction perspective.* New York: Academic Press.

Tori, C.D. (1978). A smoking satiation procedure with reduced medical risk. *Journal of Clinical Psychology, 34,* 574–577.

Van Dixhoorn, J., De Loos, J., & Duivenvoorden, H.J. (1983). Contribution of relaxation technique training to the rehabilitation of myocardial infarction patients. *Psychotherapy and Psychosomatics, 40,* 137–147.

Vetter, N.J., Cay, E.L., Philip, A.E., & Stranger, R.C. (1977). Anxiety on admission to a coronary care unit. *Journal of Psychosomatic Research, 21,* 73–78.

Vickers, R. (1973). A short measure of Type A personality. Unpublished manuscript, University of Michigan, Institute for Social Research.

Vickers, R.R., Hervig, L.K., Rahe, R.H., & Rosenman, R.H. (1981). Type A behavior pattern and coping defense. *Psychosomatic Medicine, 43,* 381–396.

Volicer, B.J., & Volicer, L. (1978). Cardiovascular changes associated with stress during hospitalization. *Journal of Psychosomatic Research, 22,* 159–168.

Wadden, T.A. (1984). Relaxation therapy for essential hypertension: Specific or non-specific effects? *Journal of Psychosomatic Research, 28,* 53–61.

Wadden, T.A., Anderson, C.H., Foster, G.D., & Love, W. (1983). The Jenkins Activity Survey: Does it measure psychopathology? *Journal of Psychosomatic Research, 27,* 321–325.

Wagner, M.K., & Bragg, R.A. (1970). Comparing behavior modification approaches to habit decrement smoking. *Journal of Consulting and Clinical Psychology, 34,* 258–263.

Wagner, N.N. (1974). Sexual adjustment of cardiac patients. *British Journal of Sexual Medicine, 1,* 17–22.

Waldron, I., Zyzanski, S., Shekelle, R.B., Jenkins, C.D., & Tannenbaum, S. (1977). The coronary-prone behavior in employed men and women. *Journal of Human Stress, 3,* 2–18.

Webb, P.A. (1980). Effectiveness of patient education and psychological counseling in promoting compliance and control among hypertensive patients. *Journal of Family Practice, 10,* 1047–1055.

Weinblatt, S., Shapiro, S., Frank, C.W., & Sager, R.V. (1966). Return to work and work status following first myocardial infarction. *American Journal of Public Health, 56,* 169–185.

Weinblatt, E., Shapiro, S., & Frank, C.W. (1971). Changes in personal characteristics of men over five years following first diagnosis of coronary artery disease. *American Journal of Public Health, 61,* 831–842.

Weinblatt, E., Ruberman, W., Goldberg, J.D., Frank, C.W., Shapiro, S., & Chaudhary, B.S. (1978). Relation of education to sudden death after myocardial infarction. *New England Journal of Medicine, 299,* 60–65.

Westlund, K. (1965). Further observations on incidence of myocardial infarction in Oslo. *Journal of the Oslo City Hospital, 15,* 201–210.

Whyte, H.M. (1983). Psychological methods of lowering blood pressure. *Medical Journal of Australia,* Special Supplement, 13–16.

Wiklund, I., Sanne, H., Vedin, A., & Wilhelmsson, C. (1984). Psychosocial outcome one year after a first myocardial infarction. *Journal of Psychosomatic Research, 28,* 309–321.

Wilhelmsen, L., Wilhelmsen, C., Vedin, A., & Elmfeldt, D. (1982). Effects of infarct size, smoking, physical activity and some psychological factors on prognosis after myocardial infarction. *Advances in Cardiology, 29,* 119–125.

Willerson, J.D., Hillis, L.D., & Buja, L.M. (1982). *Ischemic heart disease: Clinical and pathophysiological aspects.* New York: Raven Press.

Willerson, J.T. & Sanders, C.A. (Eds.) (1977). *Clinical Cardiology,* New York: Grune & Stratton.

Williams, R.B., Haney, T.L., Lee, K.L., Kong, Y., Blumenthal, J.A., & Whalen, R.E. (1980). Type A behavior, hostility and coronary atherosclerosis. *Psychosomatic Medicine, 42,* 539–549.

Wisocki, P.A., & Rooney, E.J. (1974). A comparison of thought stopping and covert sensitization techniques in the treatment of smoking: A brief report. *Psychological Record, 24,* 191–192.

Witschi, J.C., Singer, M., Wu-Lee, M., & Stare, F.J. (1978). Family cooperation and effectiveness in a cholesterol-lowering diet. *Journal of American Diet Association, 72,* 384–389.

World Health Organization. (1973). Evaluation of comprehensive rehabilitative and preventive programmes for patients after acute myocardial infarction. Copenhagen: Regional Office for Europe.

World Health Organization. (1981). The cardiovascular disease programme of WHO in Europe. Copenhagen: Regional Office for Europe.

World Health Organization. (1981). *The North Karelia Project: Community control of cardiovascular diseases.* Copenhagen: Regional Office for Europe.

World Health Organization. (1981). Report of the WHO expert committee on disability, prevention and rehabilitation. *Tech. Rep. Series No. 668.*

World Health Organization. (1983). Rehabilitation and comprehensive secondary prevention after acute myocardial infarction. Copenhagen: Regional Office for Europe.

Wright, J., Wood, B., & Hale, G. (1981). Evaluation of group versus individual nutrition education in overweight patients with myocardial infarction. *Australian New Zealand Journal of Medicine, 11,* 497–501.

Wrzesniewski, K. (1975). The development of a scale for assessing attitudes towards illness in patients experiencing a myocardial infarction. *Social Science and Medicine, 14,* 127–132.

Wrzesniewski, K. (1977). Anxiety and rehabilitation after myocardial infarction. *Psychotherapy and Psychosomatics, 27,* 41–46.

Yarian, R. (1976). The efficacy of electromyographic biofeedback training as a method of deep muscle relaxation for college students displaying either coronary or non-coronary prone behavior patterns. Unpublished manuscript, University of Maryland.

Yates, A.J. (1970). *Behavior Therapy.* New York: Wiley.

Yates, A.J. (1975). *Theory and practice in behavior therapy.* New York: Wiley.

Zacest, R., Barrow, C.G., O'Halloran, M.W., & Wilson, L.L. (1981). Relationship of psychological factors to failure of antihypertensive drug treatment. *Australian New Zealand Journal of Medicine, 11,* 501–507.

Zyzanski, S.J. (1978). Coronary-prone behavior pattern and coronary heart disease: Epidemiological evidence. In T.M. Dembroski, S.M. Weiss, J.L. Shields, Suzanne G. Haynes, M. Feinleib (Eds.), *Coronary-prone behavior.* New York: Springer-Verlag.

Zyzanski, S.J., & Jenkins, C.D. (1970). Basic dimensions within the coronary-prone behavior pattern. *Journal of Chronic Diseases, 22,* 781–792.

Zyzanski, S.J., Jenkins, C.D., Ryan, T.J., Flessas, A., & Everist, M. (1976). Psychological correlates of coronary angiographic findings. *Archives of Internal Medicine, 136,* 1234–1237.

Author Index

Subject Index